▲ Your six-month-old  baby refuses to relate to anyone except you. She turns [...] ers and screams if anyo [...]

▲ You try to convince [...] the other kids in the sandbox, but he simply shakes his head and closes his eyes.

▲ You never considered your confident, boisterous nine-year-old shy. But suddenly he withdraws from all his favorite activities and starts following you like a shadow.

▲ Your eleven-year-old daughter is a gifted athlete and a great team player. She is outgoing on the field, but off the field she has no friends and can't connect with others.

▲ Your seventh-grader is terrified of eating in the cafeteria and hides in the bathroom or goes to the nurse during lunchtime.

Shyness is a common problem among children, but its results are quite painful and harmful for everyone. The good news is that shyness *can* be overcome. Now parents can find practical, proven, hands-on solutions for all types of shyness in . . .

THE SHY CHILD

THE SHY CHILD

Helping Children Triumph over Shyness

Ward Kent Swallow, Ph.D.

with Laurie Halse Anderson

Produced by the Philip Lief Group, Inc.

WARNER BOOKS

A Time Warner Company

Copyright © 2000 by Philip Lief Group Inc.
All rights reserved.

Warner Books, Inc., 1271 Avenue of the Americas, New York, NY 10020
Visit our Web site at www.twbookmark.com

Ⓦ A Time Warner Company

Printed in the United States of America

First Printing: March 2000

10 9 8 7 6 5 4 3 2

Library of Congress Cataloging-in-Publication Data

Swallow, Ward K.
     The shy child : helping children truimph over shyness / Ward K. Swallow.
        p. cm.
     ISBN 0-446-67499-0
     1. Bashfulness in children. 2. Child rearing. I. Title.

     BF723.B3 S83 2000   99-054872
     649'.1—dc21

Book design by Nancy Singer
Cover design by Rachel McClain
Cover photo by Renzo Mancini/Image Bank

To Sarah

CONTENTS

ACKNOWLEDGMENTS

I wish to extend a special thank you to Catherine Peck and Laurie Anderson for their support of this project. I also wish to express my appreciation to my parents, George and Jolene Swallow, for modeling the importance of helping others. To my mentors, Foster Secrest and Donald Kinsley, Ph.D., I express my deepest gratitude. Lastly, thank you Kelly for your unconditional support for all of my endeavors.

THE SHY CHILD

Part One

UNDERSTANDING SHYNESS IN CHILDREN

Chapter 1

IT'S NOT JUST A PHASE: RECOGNIZING THE SHY CHILD

When your three-year-old's teacher reports that he has rarely spoken during the first weeks of preschool and then says, "But don't worry, he seems perfectly happy," you spend the night worrying anyway.

When you invite a child over to play with your four-year-old daughter, and she refuses to come out of her room and greet the visitor, you are angry, embarrassed, and worried. It has happened before. Then, when her guest leaves, your daughter emerges as her usual, happy self, dancing around the house, full of smiles—and hardly the image of a shy child.

When your daughter reaches the age of twelve and still won't answer an adult's friendly questions directly, looking instead to you to answer for her, you say to yourself, "She should have outgrown this shyness by now." Should you get professional help?

All parents worry about their children, but the parents of shy children take on an extra burden of concern. They fear their children's shyness will hinder personal development and limit their potential for fulfillment. They wonder if they have done something to cause the shyness. Day by day, they agonize along with their children when social situations loom.

It is perfectly normal to worry about your shy child. Shyness *can* interfere with a child's growth and development, school performance, friendships, and social experiences. Unless issues surrounding shyness are addressed in childhood, they are often carried into adulthood, where they can lead to loneliness, self-doubt, and even despair.

If you are shy yourself, you understand how hard it is to face a world filled with people who seem socially confident. If you are not a shy person, you may be baffled by your child's behavior. If there are siblings in the family who are not shy, it is hard to avoid comparing the children. What can you do?

You are a good parent. You love your child deeply and are trying to find the best way to raise her in a challenging world. You are in good company. There are millions more shy children in the world than you ever dreamed of, and their parents—like you—are seeking guidance and support. The following chapters are designed to offer you guidelines—based on clinical observations of shy children—about what works and what doesn't work when helping children come to terms with shyness.

Successfully parenting a shy child will require you to understand the nature of shyness, to respect your child's individuality, and to provide a bridge between your child's interior self and the outside world. That bridge can be constructed from the coping skills described in this book, and you are the best person to present them to your child. The rewards will be great. Not only will your child gain confidence and courage that will carry him into adulthood, but by working closely with your child and confronting shyness together, you can form a lasting bond that many parents only dream of having with their children.

FACING SHYNESS

Parents can help children come to terms with shyness best if they first overcome their own biases and fears about its impact on their children's lives. So let's face those biases and fears squarely.

We cannot ignore the possible consequences of unattended shyness. There is not doubt that it has the potential to harm children in terms of their development. If a shy child is allowed to turn away from the world, if he never learns how to take control of the anxiety that paralyzes him or master the self-consciousness that plagues him, there is a good chance he will grow into a shy adult.

Shy adults who do not have good coping skills are vulnerable. They tend not to excel in the work world. They stay in jobs that are below their skill level and that allow them to escape dealing with other people. They often are loners. They watch others' apparent social grace and wonder why they cannot interact with such ease. Those who marry, often marry the first person with whom they have a significant relationship. Shy adults can even develop anxiety disorders or become severely depressed.

These outcomes are not inevitable, however. The low self-esteem that often accompanies sadness and vulnerability in shy adults is largely the result not of shyness itself but of societal attitudes toward shy behavior, of early parental reactions, and of a spoken or unspoken assumption that there is something abnormal in being shy. By examining these attitudes, reactions, and assumptions, we can arrive at an understanding of what shyness is not, and then get a clear idea of what shyness *is*.

How Our Culture Views Shyness

American culture celebrates the outspoken, the bold, the brash, and the brave. We honor people who are willing to stand up for themselves, voice their opinions, and bring attention to their causes. We admire celebrities who bask in the limelight, full of self-assurance and confidence.

Shyness is typically viewed as a thing to be conquered. Americans applaud the athlete who performs after crying in fear. We cheer for the actress who confesses to stage fright, but somehow pulls herself together and gives a stellar performance. It is acceptable to be a *formerly* shy person, as long as you have figured out how to vanquish your native bashfulness.

Gender expectations complicate the American view of shyness. It seems somehow more acceptable for girls to be shy. "Quiet girls are good girls" is a message that we still receive. But shy girls sometimes "fall between the cracks" in school settings and social situations because their teachers and peers see them as self-contained children who do not need attention. Consequently, they are less likely to be called on in school, and, even though their grades may be good, they are less likely to receive demonstrative, public praise.

Ironically, while shyness is more acceptable in girls than in boys, when girls reach adulthood they find that aggressiveness and attention-seeking behavior are culturally desirable in the working world, while the diffidence that kept them on good terms with adults is detrimental to career advancement. In other words, for girls and women, what was cute at age six, may be debilitating at thirty-six.

Shy boys often raise red flags for adults more quickly than girls do because boys are not, culturally speaking, expected to be quiet and self-contained. A boy who does not draw attention to himself is more likely than a girl to have attention thrust upon him by a well-meaning teacher or not-so-well-meaning schoolyard peers. Shy boys are sometimes tormented and bullied. Adult attempts to draw them out, though, often lead to embarrassment and further withdrawal.

Our society values group participation, a willingness to enter in, to get involved. When a member of a group hangs back and seems unwilling to join in an activity, we sometimes assume it is a choice she is making. Shyness is sometimes mislabeled as snobbishness. In fact, while shy people usually feel like they are being left out of a group, they are often surprised if they learn that the people in the in group feel it is they who have been rejected, rather than the other way around.

For the shy child, however, remaining outside the group is rarely a choice at first. Primarily because of inordinate self-consciousness, shy boys and girls simply do not know how to initiate conversation or find their place among their peers. Since it is ultimately more comfortable to refuse to join in than to risk embarrassment by speaking up, it is not uncommon for a shy child to convince herself that she is making a conscious choice to remain aloof, which only adds to the impression that she thinks herself "above the crowd." Thus begins a negative cycle of social exclusion.

Parental Responses to Childhood Shyness

Given the cultural tendency to value outspokenness over re-serve, it is easy to see how shyness comes to be seen as an enemy that must be defeated. One way parents respond to this view is to take the attitude that if the kid would just toughen up, he wouldn't be so shy. It is the "throw them in the pool and they'll figure out how to swim" school of thought. Some children do respond to this approach, but most don't. Forcing a child to fight against his natural tendencies can be disastrous.

The opposite parental response is also common, which is to swoop in and rescue the socially awkward child; to speak up for her when she becomes tongue-tied; or to remove her from a situation that is causing her distress. But trying to overpro-tect a child risks teaching her that she can avoid difficult cir-cumstances, with the consequence that she will never learn the necessary skills to become a competent adult in today's so-ciety.

As the parent of a shy child, you do need to monitor your child's comfort level in school and play situations. There will be times when you need to shield him to prevent genuine trauma, and there will be times when you need to leave him to his own devices. By learning to understand what motivates shy behavior, you can accurately gauge which action to take at a given time. All along the way, the most effective action you can take will be to offer your child a clear, realistic picture of himself and his motivations, along with the coping skills he needs to become comfortable dealing with the world within the context of his shy personality.

Shy tendencies are not your child's enemy. Many fine qualities that are as crucial to the smooth functioning of our society as outgoingness and self-advancement go hand in hand with shyness. A keen sense of observation, empathy for others, self-awareness, and a rich interior life are the hallmarks of adults who began life as shy children. By recognizing them as assets, you can help your child learn to *use* them to advantage.

Shyness Is Not Abnormal

Shy children tend to think they are different from their peers. Nothing could be further from the truth. Studies show that 20 percent of children are born shy and another 20 percent develop shyness before adulthood. With 40 percent of the population identified as shy, it is clear that shyness is not an aberration or a problem faced by a small group. Shyness is a personality style shared by millions.

All children exhibit shyness at some point in their lives. Even the more outgoing baby will occasionally turn away from strangers, and a normally confident child may quake in front of a group. A disruption in family life such as a move or divorce can temporarily cause an ebullient child to become withdrawn. Situational or reactive shyness can be seen as a defense mechanism, a survival technique, a necessary hanging back to watch and wait and make sure the coast is clear before moving on.

A nonshy person may *feel* shy in unfamiliar surroundings or when confronted by someone who makes him feel inferior. We have a rich vocabulary to describe our feelings in these situations. We get butterflies in the stomach, a frog in the throat, or cold feet. We are in a sweat, in a dither, or in a tizzy. The language is colorful, but the emotions are wretched. It is important to remember that everyone has these feelings at one time or another. Consider the following situations in which shy behavior is normal in children.

- *Meeting new people.* Being forced to interact with people they are not familiar with produces predictable shy behavior in children whether they are genuinely shy or not. Children will cast their eyes to the ground, mumble, hide, or even ignore the new person. It is an awkward moment. As flustered as the parent may feel, the child feels worse. She doesn't know what to say or do, and there is no place to hide.

- *Speaking in front of a group.* Some kids love to perform; they were born to be at center stage. They thrive on the sensation of having all eyes focused on them, of holding the attention of an entire group. There are some shy children who also have this ability, a paradox that will be examined later. (See "Shy Extroverts" in Chapter 2 and "Interest Groups" in Chapter 9.) Yet most children respond to the prospect of having to speak in front of others with alarm. Their throats close. Their hands sweat. Their hearts pound. They imagine the worst things that could happen: They'll trip on the way to the podium; they'll drop their notes; their pants will fall down. It would be funny if it weren't so painful.

- *A new environment.* Places can become comfortable just like an old pair of blue jeans or a blanket. A child who moves in the familiar orbit of home and school, with side trips to friends' houses or the mall, doesn't even stop to think about these places. They just are there. But put a child in an unfamiliar setting and watch what happens. She will look for something familiar or a face she recognizes. She may pull into herself a bit. Many children are wary in new settings. The first day of school, a new house, an unfamiliar bus stop, all are likely to cause shy behavior.

The nonshy child will experience sensations of fear or social reticence briefly. After a few minutes of watching an unfamiliar child stand awkwardly in her foyer, the nonshy child will ask her guest to play and off they'll go. The nonshy child will survive reading her report to the whole class and will probably be comfortable the next time she has to do it. She will adjust to her new playground, or school, or house, quickly making it her own.

Not so for the shy child. For a chronically shy person, the defense mechanism remains in place for a much longer time, and the shy child reacts with wariness in almost every new situation. Often they do not attribute their success in life to their actions. The shy child meets a new person and can be flooded with fear and anxiety that does not go away quickly. Called on to read a report, she is likely to have physical reactions severe enough to make her feel genuinely sick. Adjusting to a new setting can take months. Children don't have the ability to articulate their feelings clearly or explore the rationale behind their emotions. They just turn to their parents with tears in their eyes and feel very, very different.

It is at such times that you, as the parent of a shy child, can remember that shyness *does* make a child feel different, but shy behavior is not abnormal. It is perfectly ordinary and normal for your child to react the way she does.

Shyness *Is* a Personality Style

Shyness is not a disorder. Shyness is not a disability. Shyness is not cause for parental despair or societal intolerance.

Tape this to your bathroom mirror: *Shyness is a personality style*.

Your child is not doomed to a life on the fringes of society. He can develop confidence. He can learn to interpret realistically what others think of him. He can make friends and move comfortably in a social circle. He can do all this, not in spite of his shyness, but within the context of his shy personality.

Your attitude toward shyness affects your child's vision of herself. If you think that shy children are weak characters, your child will perceive herself as weak and undeserving. If you are highly anxious about your child's shyness, she is likely to think that she has some kind of illness or disorder. If, on the other hand, you see shyness as just one part of your child's multifaceted personality, then she will accept it herself and, most important, remain open to your ideas about how to cope.

So let's repeat one more time: *Shyness is a personality style*.

Shyness is nothing to be afraid of. By understanding the nature of shyness and society's reaction to it, you can begin the task of *supporting* your shy child as she learns skills that will give her a stronger awareness of herself. You can be instrumental in convincing her that she is capable of taking charge of her actions and reactions. To begin the process, it's time to take a closer look at your child. How can you tell if he or she is truly shy?

IS MY CHILD SHY?

Shy children share certain predictable characteristics. If you have never talked about your child's shyness with another parent, do it this week. There is generally a great sense of camaraderie among parents of shy children. It can be tremendously comforting to learn that your child is not alone. Neither are you.

If you think your child is shy, read over the descriptions below. Do any of these stories sound familiar?

AVOIDING EYE CONTACT

Nicole's mother was at her wit's end. It felt as if Nicole had been crying from the minute she was born, with only brief breaks for a nap or nursing. The doctor said the baby had colic, the grandmothers shook their heads, and the neighbors all offered useless advice. By the time Nicole was six months old, she had outgrown the colic, but she still screamed if anyone other than her mother picked her up. As long as it was just the two of them, Nicole would coo, giggle, and behave like any other baby. As soon as they neared other people, Nicole would become quiet. If anyone approached her stroller, Nicole would turn her head to the side, refusing to look at anyone who was not her mother. If the stranger touched her, or stayed in front of the stroller, she would erupt into screams, and her mother would have to take her home, exhausted, confused, and worried. Her baby couldn't even look at another person.

Avoiding eye contact is one way that shy children reduce the tension of being around others. It buffers the intensity of the experience. Because eye contact is so personal, others might interpret a shy person's looking away as a sign of discomfort, shame, fear, dishonesty, or an unwillingness to establish intimacy. In a child, it is usually a signal she is feeling vulnerable. As the story of Nicole illustrates, this kind of avoidance can begin in infancy.

WHEN ALL ELSE FAILS, DO NOTHING

Brandon's parents thought that joining a Cub Scout troop would help him make friends. They hoped that the smaller group of boys and shared interests would make him more comfortable. He didn't show any enthusiasm when he was told about the new activity, but he didn't complain either. Since Brandon had previously absolutely refused to join the soccer team, his parents thought his lack of protest was a good sign.

Months later Brandon's mother received a phone call from another mother in the troop who was looking for information about the wooden race cars the Cub Scouts were making. Brandon's mother was confused; she had never heard about the race cars. The other mother filled her in on the details. All the Scouts were supposed to be working on their pinewood racers at home. A competitive derby was scheduled in two weeks. Didn't Brandon's mother get the notes?

Brandon didn't want to talk about it. He wasn't exactly sure what to do, and he was too uncomfortable to talk to his scoutmaster about it. He hadn't shown his mother the note because he knew she would make him talk to the scoutmaster. Brandon could not explain why talking to the scoutmaster was so hard, he just didn't want to do it. It was easier not to say anything.

When she asked, the scoutmaster told her that Brandon never joined in with the other boys. He sat alone twisting his neckerchief and watched the others. He seemed to enjoy working on badges that he could do alone, but the other boys complained about his lack of cooperation in joint projects.

Brandon's mother was at a total loss. How could Brandon just sit there? Why was it so hard for him to ask for help or participate?

When a child hides or cries in the face of a new situation, you have a shot at identifying the emotion he is wrestling with. But what if he just sits motionless and gives no sign that he's aware of what is going on around him? Have you ever tried to introduce your child to a friend of yours, only to have him ignore both of you entirely? What is he thinking?

It will help to remember that the shy child is always feeling something, and he is probably tuned in to everything. But shy children experience a great deal of "self-talk," a running interior dialogue that can interfere with his immediate response to the outside world. So though it appears to you that your child is sitting there doing nothing, his mind is, in fact, alive with activity. He is imagining all kinds of scenarios, and he is left feeling unsure of which one he should choose. In moments of severe shyness, this interior dialogue can seem to paralyze a child, leading to negative feelings of self-doubt and even shame. (The concept of self-talk and its influence on shyness will be discussed at length in Chapter 2.)

THE TEMPER TANTRUMS OF AN ANGEL

Leeanne was the kind of child that people stared at. She was beautiful, with large sparkling eyes and a shy smile. She was not outgoing, but calmly did what her second-grade teacher asked her to do without complaint. She had one good friend, Emily, with whom she played every day after school. Emily's mother, Barbara, was enchanted by Leeanne. The little girl was neat, organized, and polite.

Leeanne's mother, Sue, called Barbara one evening in a desperate voice. Could they meet for coffee? There was something she had to talk about.

Sue was still near tears when she arrived at the coffee shop. She said she didn't know what to do next, where to turn. She was even thinking of psychotherapy for her eight-year-old. She explained that Leeanne's temper tantrums had been getting worse and worse. Leeanne had always had a short fuse at home, but now the whole family was walking on eggshells. When a crayon broke, she threw the box on the floor and stomped on it. When Sue told her she couldn't watch television until she picked up her clothes, she became defiant and went to bed crying before she would do what she was told.

Barbara was shocked. At her house Leeanne always behaved perfectly. Why would she throw such hideous tantrums at home?

Shy children sometimes experience spontaneous, blind rages that adults interpret as "temper tantrums." Parents are understandably baffled when such strange emotions come over a child who normally appears self-contained and content. What they don't realize is that children who are in school or day care spend most of their waking hours in situations that provoke anxiety for those who are shy. Think for a moment about what it feels like to be terribly anxious: sweaty palms, palpitating heart, nervous jitters. What if you felt like that many times a day, every day? Children tend to act out their emotions.

Once home—and safe—a child who experiences that level of anxiety needs release, and sometimes the smallest incident can set her off, as in the case of Leeanne.

YEP. NOPE. DUNNO.

Alexander's parents were increasingly worried. He had learned to speak normally and could be quite verbal if he was in the right mood. Playing alone in his room with his action figures, he talked a mile a minute. But in third grade, he grew more and more reluctant to talk with his parents or anyone else.

His parents had his hearing tested, even though they suspected it would prove nothing. He could hear perfectly, he just didn't like to talk. His teacher reported that he played alone at recess but sometimes sat with one boy at lunch. If she called on him to read an answer from his homework, he would speak. If she asked him his opinion or for an answer during a class discussion, he just shook his head. His grandparents were worried too. Alexander could rarely manage more than "Hello" on the telephone. Was he becoming rebellious and troubled, or was he just shy?

Many children are reluctant to fill parents in on their lives away from home, especially as they get into adolescence. But shy children are notorious from the start for answering in monosyllables when asked direct questions. Sometimes, if they get the idea that their parents are concerned about their level of participation at school, the question "What did you do at school today" may be met with silence meant to hide the fact that they didn't do much.

Short answers might also be a result of the self-talk going on in the shy child's mind. Perhaps she's going over the many possible ways to answer a question and gauging her parents' possible reaction to each. Indecision may cause her to take the easy way out by saying simply, "nope."

Shy children often have talkative siblings who seem to them to take up all the available talking time. The child who needs to consider carefully the words he will choose to speak, gets used to the fact that he might never get a word in edge-wise. Many shy children are only too happy to let older, or even younger, more outgoing siblings do all the talking. It lets them off the hook.

Grilling a shy child can lead to balkiness. Asking him how he feels is usually futile, because he may not *know*, or be able to express how he feels. On the other hand, when you, as parent, ask simple yes-or-no questions of your child, you invite monosyllabic answers. Adults have to walk a fine line here, and more will be said later on strategies to draw out the shy child.

SILENT IN THE CLASSROOM

Robert's parents knew that their son was considered one of the "quiet" boys, but it had never affected his schoolwork until fifth grade. Robert had one good friend and seemed content and well adjusted. He was not boisterous. He did not run around with the group of neighborhood kids who played kickball and street hockey. But he and his buddy enjoyed watching cartoons together or hunting for salamanders. And Robert always brought home good grades.

The phone call from Robert's fifth-grade teacher came as a surprise. The teacher asked for a meeting. Robert's grades after the first six weeks of school were alarmingly inconsistent. They looked nothing like his performance in fourth grade.

Robert's written reports were all Bs and As. His artwork was creative. But his test grades were extremely low and he refused to participate in class. What could be the problem?

His parents' concern grew when they talked to their son. He didn't seem to have an answer. He shrugged and squirmed under their questions. Fifth grade wasn't harder than fourth grade, but it was different. He said he hated the tests; they made him feel sick. His best friend wasn't in his class this year. He felt like the other children were making fun of him all the time, though he couldn't provide any examples of this.

Robert's parents thought their son was just being lazy. They threatened to ground him until his grades came back up and he behaved in class. Robert grew angry with them and shouted—nobody understood him. He just wanted to go back to fourth grade when everything was perfect.

The classroom can be a terribly intimidating setting for a shy child, particularly in a school district that does not keep the same group of children together from year to year. Oral reports and group projects designed to encourage social skills only add stress. With classes of twenty-five or thirty students, teachers don't have the time they need to understand every individual. Those teachers who are not alert to the ways of the shy child may view him as a reluctant learner, or even as someone with learning differences.

DON'T MAKE ME ASK

Twelve-year-old Victoria opened the cheeseburger box and sighed. The lady who worked at the McDonald's had not given her extra ketchup. She bit the inside of her cheek. She loved ketchup. She really wanted more. She looked across the table at her ten-year-old sister, Amy.

Amy shook her head. "No way," she said. "I always have to get your stuff. Go up and ask her yourself. She's not going to hurt you."

Victoria watched Amy dig into her lunch. Why was it so easy for Amy to talk to strangers? It had been this way since they were little. Amy had always been completely comfortable doing things that Victoria thought were impossible. When they shopped for hair scrunchies, Amy would ask the clerk for the color Victoria needed because Victoria was too embarrassed. When Victoria was desperate for a bathroom while they were playing at a friend's house, little Amy had asked the friend's mother where it was. And Amy always, always went back for ketchup or napkins or a second order of fries when they went to McDonald's. It had become something of a family joke.

Their father watched Victoria shred her napkin as she agonized over the ketchup decision. He knew she would end up eating her fries without it, and he was torn. He hated to see her unhappy, even over such a little thing. But she had to learn to ask for simple things like this. How would she survive college or ever get a job if she needed her little sister to do the talking for her?

Asking for help makes the shy child feel more vulnerable than usual. It is not uncommon for a shy child to avoid using the telephone for years. Paying for purchases at a store's cash register, often a thrilling rite of passage for a nonshy child, can remain out of the question for a shy child until well into her teens. Parents are baffled at the lengths to which a child will go in order to avoid having to speak up for herself in simple situations.

RED CHEEKS, SWEATY PALMS, AND DRY MOUTH

Leslie had practiced her flute for months to prepare for the state competition. She was extremely proud of her reputation as the best flute player in her middle school. Her parents were happy that she had made a place for herself in the band and now had a small group of friends. Music was one way their shy daughter could reach out to other people. However, playing solo had always been a problem for her.

The day of the competition, Leslie wanted to ride the bus with the rest of the band. Her parents followed behind in the van, commenting on how much she had grown and what a confident fourteen-year-old she was becoming. They could see her laughing with her friends. But when Leslie stepped off the bus, she looked like a different person. No more giggling. The other band members were nervous too, but Leslie lagged far behind the group as they walked down the hall.

Each competitor had to perform in the band room in front of one judge and an assistant. When Leslie's name was called, she flushed bright red from her hairline to her neck. She fumbled with her music. She hesitated at the door. Her heart was pounding and she could feel her underarms getting wet. She forced herself through the door and set her music on the stand with shaking hands. The judge nodded. Leslie raised the flute to her mouth and . . . nothing. She couldn't blow. Her tongue felt as if it had swollen to fill her mouth completely. The flute slid under her fingers from the sweat on her hands. Her lips fused to the mouthpiece. She couldn't even get a squeak out of her instrument. She was in a complete panic and didn't know what to do next. [Stage fright may have a specific relationship to shyness.]

The notion of the "fight or flight syndrome" has become familiar to most of us. In tense situations, our bodies prepare to confront the source of our fear or to run away as fast as we can. Our pupils enlarge so we can see better, our hearing becomes more acute, our muscles tense to deal with the challenge, blood pumps to provide more oxygen to brain cells, and heart and respiration rates increase. These physiological responses are useful when hunting wild boars and escaping muggers. They get in the way when the "threat" is something as harmless as a band competition.

MY STOMACH HURTS

Derek's parents were so concerned about his constant stomachaches that they took him to their family doctor. Was their high school sophomore developing an ulcer?

Derek hated all the attention. Why couldn't everyone just leave him alone? His parents insisted. Derek complained all the time about his aching stomach; the night before a test he could barely choke down dinner.

The doctor found nothing wrong and the specialist hinted that Derek was trying to get out of doing schoolwork. The entire family was insulted by that. Derek was a solid student who wasn't trying to get away with anything. During the long trip home from the doctor's, Derek admitted that he usually went to the nurse's office during lunch. It was quiet there and he didn't feel as if everyone was staring at him. Hearing this, his father lost his temper. How could Derek be afraid of the lunchroom?

The parents called the school and insisted that Derek be forbidden from using the nurse's office as a hideout. Derek didn't say anything at the time, but two weeks later the school called. Derek had been absent several days and did not have a signed excuse note. Did his parents know he was cutting class?

Physiological responses such as stomachaches or the general complaint of "I don't feel good" are also tied to anxiety in shy children. All children have used these excuses at one time or another to get out of doing something they don't want to do. For many children, physiological problems are a genuine response to anxiety. The stomachache on the day of the oral report or the school dance is not imagined; it is real. But it is caused by stress, not a virus, and it sometimes becomes for the child a reliable way to avoid embarrassing situations.

NOBODY LIKES ME

The explosion came out of nowhere. Ashley's mother went in to say good night to her eighth-grade daughter, and the girl burst into sobs. She clung to her mother for the better part of an hour, crying so hard it brought tears to her mother's eyes.

Ashley couldn't explain what was wrong at first. Her mother made them both a cup of hot chocolate and found a fresh box of tissues. Ashley was reluctant to admit what was wrong, but she finally said it, "I have no friends!" and burst into tears again.

Ashley's mother held her. "Of course you have friends," she said. She listed the names of the girls Ashley sat with at lunch, the kids who called for help with homework. "You are always talking about this person or that person. You know everyone in your school. You're just feeling oversensitive; you need a good night's sleep."

Ashley drew away from her mother. "Nobody knows who I am. Nobody knows what I feel inside or what I like and what I want to do. Everybody is so superficial it makes me sick. I feel like I'm the only person on the planet who thinks these things. You're no better than them. You don't understand either."

Shy children do not always interpret social signals properly. They often feel that a situation is awkward when, for others in the room, it is not. You might hear your shy child complain that "Everyone was staring at me" or "Nobody ever talks to me." Their hyperawareness of negative feelings can lead them to ignore positive social signals they get from other children. They may indeed have friendships, but they tend to discount them, particularly when they are feeling stressed or left out.

Assessing Your Child's Shyness

How does your child's shyness show itself in his daily life? Is his shy behavior only temporary—the result of a developmental shift that has left him feeling awkward? Or is shyness an integral part of his personality? The following informal assessment provides questions you can ask yourself about your child that will give you some insight into areas of his life where shyness may intrude now or may cause him problems later. Once you are ready to begin to address his shyness according to the recommendations in this book, this assessment will help you zero in on the behaviors that most need attention.

As children come to understand their shyness, they will likely begin to respond to social situations differently. You can return to this assessment every six months or so to see whether or not you think your child's behavior has changed either as a result of work you have done together or as a result of natural developmental changes.

After each question, circle the answer that most accurately describes your child's behavior. Notice which questions you answer by circling "always" or "frequently." These will help clarify for you the areas where your child's shyness may be causing him difficulty now, or may cause him anxiety later.

1. Is your child uncomfortable playing with other children of the same age he does not know?

   Always   Frequently   Occasionally   Never

2. If your child fearful of new situations?

   Always   Frequently   Occasionally   Never

3. Does your child demonstrate significant signs of anxiety when asked to speak in front of a group?

   Always   Frequently   Occasionally   Never

4. Does your child avoid safe situations where he would have to interact with strangers?

   Always   Frequently   Occasionally   Never

5. Does your child routinely make incorrect assumptions about the way others view him?

   Always   Frequently   Occasionally   Never

6. Does your child (six years or older) have temper tantrums or refuse to leave a family member when it is time for school, or in other separation situations?

Always   Frequently   Occasionally   Never

7. Given a choice, would your child prefer to play alone?

Always   Frequently   Occasionally   Never

8. When confronted with new social situations, does your child experience physical signs of anxiety such as stomachaches, headaches, trembling, sweating, blushing, shortness of breath, nausea, or dizziness that are not connected to an illness?

Always   Frequently   Occasionally   Never

9. Does your child worry excessively about upcoming events or activities?

Always   Frequently   Occasionally   Never

10. Does your child freeze in normal social situations, not knowing how to act or what is expected?

Always   Frequently   Occasionally   Never

11. Does your child need recovery time alone after a social situation?

    Always   Frequently   Occasionally   Never

12. Does anxiety interfere with your child's schoolwork?

    Always   Frequently   Occasionally   Never

13. Does your child avoid pleasurable activities that would put him in contact with unfamiliar people?

    Always   Frequently   Occasionally   Never

14. Does your child overreact with feelings of shame or low self-worth after social interactions?

    Always   Frequently   Occasionally   Never

15. Does your child depend on family members to act as a constant buffer, communicating his needs and wants to strangers?

    Always   Frequently   Occasionally   Never

The Shyness Spectrum

Shy children will move across the shyness spectrum and back again depending on their developmental age, family situation, and other external influences such as friendships and relationships with school. Your child may be confident at one age and painfully shy at another. You may also notice that she is confident in some situations or with some trusted friends but seems terrified in other situations or with a different set of children around her. One child may be shy only in public, while another may experience a deeper-rooted shyness that affects family relationships. Children tend to show stronger shy tendencies when they reach developmental milestones. Moving up from elementary to middle school or from middle school to high school can cause a child who has previously learned to override shyness to revert to his former reticence.

Understanding where your child is on the spectrum can help you decide what kind of support she needs. Based on your answers to the assessment above and the descriptions below, you should be able to assess the level of your child's shyness. As the child's parent, you are the best person to evaluate how much help she needs in coming to terms with her shyness. The most important question to ask along the way is: Does shyness interfere with my child's ability to develop socially, emotionally, or intellectually?

Moderately Shy. A moderately shy child is well adjusted academically and socially, but appears quiet relative to peers and siblings. His teachers may describe him as "reserved." He has one or two good friends and is generally well thought of by his acquaintances. He prefers to work independently instead of in groups, and he is quite happy to be alone. If he doesn't have enough time alone, he may grow restless and irritable.

Moderately shy children become most anxious when they are forced into social situations over which they have no control. Their anxiety becomes apparent too when well-laid plans

go awry. For example, a child may be bold enough to participate in the class play, during which he feels he knows exactly
what will happen. But if on the night of the dress rehearsal his
costume doesn't work out as he expected, or some other
change makes him feel out of control, he may find his confidence wavering significantly. Parents may notice that such behaviors are more likely to flare up when their child is tired.

Moderately shy children generally find it easy to understand what shyness is, they accept the fact that other children
are more outgoing, and they tend to be more comfortable
with their personalities.

Strongly Shy. A child who is strongly shy shows a number of
avoidance behaviors. She goes out of her way to avoid being
around people she does not know well. She has a hard time
looking people in the eye. She has a number of physical reactions to stressful situations such as tense stomach, flushing,
and sweaty palms.

The strongly shy child is lacking in confidence and is socially anxious. She may appear to be withdrawn, unresponsive,
and uncommunicative. She often daydreams, since living in a
world of imagination is preferable to facing an unpleasant reality. She sometimes allows herself to be placed in an anxiety-
producing situation, but then fails to follow through. For
example she may accept an invitation to a sleep-over at a
friend's house and then find that it is too stressful to sleep
without her family about her and ask to be taken home.

Severely Shy. The severely shy child might need professional
help. His anxiety has progressed to a disorder. He may suffer
a social phobia, panic disorder, or major depression. A social
phobia can be expressed as agoraphobia, the fear of leaving

the home and a fear of open spaces. However, this disorder is thought to be more often motivated by a need to protect someone in the house than by apprehension toward the outside world.

Parents should trust their instincts about children who are severely shy from birth or seem suddenly to become severely shy. Children have a hard time distinguishing between normal anxiety and phobias, so even if your child denies any problem or avoids any discussion about it, you will want to gather as much information about his behavior as you can. If your child wanders to this far edge of the shyness spectrum, seek professional help.

THE GOOD NEWS

Realizing that your child is shy can be disappointing or even frightening. You know that life can be difficult for a shy person in our culture. You fear that shyness will get in the way of her happiness. However, although there are no magic wands you can wave that will make a timid child brave, there is plenty for you to do to help your child use her style to her best advantage.

You have already taken the first steps by acknowledging and accepting your child's shy tendencies. Now you are ready to understand what is going on inside your child—what confusing emotions make it difficult for her to find her own way. Once you understand her better, and understand the causes of shyness and its impact on the family, then you can begin to assemble the tools that will help her make the necessary adjustments to face the world with courage and confidence.

Chapter 2

THE INFLUENCE OF SELF-TALK ON THE SHY CHILD

A mother tries to convince her son to join the other children in the sandbox. "They're nice," she says. "They want you to play with them. You'll be fine." But her son only shakes his head and closes his eyes.

In the lobby of a dance studio a confused father argues with his daughter. "But you wanted me to sign you up for lessons," he reminds her. "Why can't you just go in there? Nobody is staring at you. This is ridiculous." The daughter says nothing. She cannot stop the tears of embarrassment washing down her red cheeks.

What happens in the minds of shy children to transform everyday situations into dramatic, terrifying experiences? What are they thinking? Parents of shy children have all reached the point where they would give anything to be able to see the world through their shy child's eyes.

This chapter will show you how your shy child interprets

the world. You may be surprised. Shy children experience the world differently than nonshy children—and quite differently from adults. Understanding how your child perceives events and processes information to produce negative self-talk is the first step to knowing how you can help him.

THE CONCEPT OF SELF-TALK

Developments in behavioral psychology in the last fifteen years have given us simple, practical tools to use with our children. One of the most powerful new concepts is the regulation of self-talk. Self-talk describes the ongoing conversation we hold with ourselves. Sometimes referred to as "automatic thoughts," self-talk is a constant background flow commenting on our experiences and regulating our emotional state. Self-talk can be a quiet brook when all is well, or it can flood like an angry river when we feel upset. Self-talk can be energizing, uplifting, and encouraging, or it can be destructive, humiliating, and poisonous.

Recognizing Self-Talk

We all experience self-talk, whether or not we are consciously aware of it. When you remind yourself to stop at the store on the way home from work, and later when you realize you are three blocks past the store and call yourself "stupid," you are experiencing self-talk. Automatic thoughts rush by quickly, sometimes too fast for you to sense them, but they leave behind a residue of emotion. For shy children, these emotions are often feelings of anxiety, insecurity, or anger.

What we think affects how we feel and act; automatic thoughts help direct emotion and behavior. Can you hear your self-talk? Are you secretly wondering if some traumatic incident in your child's life made her inhibited? Are you worried that your spouse thinks your concern for your child is overblown? What are the anxieties, the messages creeping into your conscious thought? Are they positive, such as "You are awesome!" or negative, such as "You loser"?

Self-talk guides our behavior. Some aspects of self-talk are what we refer to as our good conscience: the social rules that tell us what is and what is not acceptable to do. One of the developmental tasks of childhood is to take the rules of life presented to us by our elders and internalize them, transform them into our self-talk so we can regulate ourselves and fit into society. A two-year-old will grab a cookie on the table, usually without hesitation, whereas a five-year-old will look around first, either to seek permission from an adult, or to see if he can sneak the cookie without being noticed. The five-year-old has absorbed the family lesson of "no cookies before dinner." This behavior-guidance aspect of automatic thoughts is the easiest to identify within ourselves, easiest to describe, and easiest to discuss with other people.

But the power of self-talk extends far beyond the conscience. Shy children experience a great deal of self-talk that can be called "social appraisal." That is, they "hear" messages that concern whatever social situation they are in, or anticipate they may be in. You have probably experienced social appraisal self-talk when you have entered a party where you didn't know anyone, and you then had to work the room. Positive social appraisal self-talk may be messages such as "I look fabulous. He is hanging on my every word. I'm going to get a job offer out of this." Negative social appraisal self-talk is easy to imagine: "They know I'm a fake. Is my zipper open? I'm boring her. I bet they fire me first thing in the morning."

People who suffer from anxiety or depression experience more negative or fearful self-talk than people who feel calm and in control of their lives. This negative self-talk feeds into a vicious, self-defeating cycle. In an anxiety-provoking situation, such as an awkward conversation at a dinner party, an anxious person will remember other times when he felt completely out of his depth. Instead of thinking of constructive things he can do or topics to talk about, he may hear self-talk in short bursts, harsh messages such as "Idiot," "You are so stupid," "You don't belong here," "They are laughing at you." This interior monologue then distorts the person's view of his situation. Sometimes, these monologues are so habitual they become outside of a person's normal awareness.

The knowledge that a negative interior monologue distorts reality is extremely important. People who suffer from negative self-talk misinterpret social situations. When a stranger glances at them, they may perceive the look as one of loathing. An innocent "How are you?" may be thought to be sarcastic or hostile. The negative emotions surrounding this social situation continue to build. The anxious person then makes bad decisions, lashing out at a friendly gesture—perhaps even overreacting physically—until, finally, he flees. The situation is filed away as another disastrous memory that will be trotted out and replayed whenever a new situation provokes anxiety and the negative self-talk kicks in again.

Positive self-talk, on the other hand, can help build confidence. Self-help programs that urge their followers to "fake it till you make it" utilize the power of positive self-talk. When you smile in an effort to raise your spirits, tell yourself everything will work out fine, or give yourself a pep talk, you employ positive self-talk.

There is a third category of self-talk that will be utilized a great deal later in this book. It is called neutral self-talk, and it involves low-key messages such as "It's okay" or "I'm fine." These neutral messages have the effect of keeping the mind in a neutral state, neither happy nor sad, and they can see a naturally anxious person through a difficult time until more distinctly positive self-talk is available.

Self-Talk in Children

Children experience as much self-talk as adults. In fact, there is evidence that children have self-talk messages even before they have language skills. Their brains are able to think about how good chocolate pudding tastes long before they can string together a sentence to ask for it. Children who have not developed language have more stimulus response connections in their brains. It is obvious that a great deal of activity is going on in their minds, activity that is mirrored in their behavior and emotions.

As spoken language emerges, usually between ten and twenty-four months, we can hear our children's self-talk messages. Young children talk to themselves, or to dolls and other toys, allowing us a valuable window into their emotional state. A girl who praises herself when she stacks her blocks shows she is proud of her accomplishment and she feels competent. As she grows up, those early messages of "Good job!" will boost her self-confidence. Conversely, a little girl who consistently calls herself "dummy" is headed toward a lifetime of internal criticism.

Some researchers have raised the intriguing suggestion that imaginary friends grow out of the automatic thoughts of children. Children will sometimes develop imaginary friends between the ages of two and one half and six years of age. These friends can seem quite real to a child, who give them physical attributes, life histories, and strong personalities. It may be that the impetus for these friends is the child's recognition of automatic thoughts; it may seem to a child that there really is someone whispering "Big boy" or "I'm afraid" in their ears.

Nonshy children often have energetic, action-oriented, risk-taking self-talk, messages such as, "Sure, I'll play with him. Who cares? Hey guys, look at me! Watch what I can do!" These children are drawn to others. They do not ruminate on what other children think of them; they simply enjoy being in the presence of and interacting with other kids.

In contrast, the shy child minutely evaluates every social step with self-talk messages. "If I take the red block, will he frown at me? Is she angry? Why did she turn her back on me?" Often the introvert analyzes everything down to the tiniest detail and remembers the smallest gesture and nuance. As the parent of a shy child, you might see your child express indifference toward others, either in words or body language, and this might be confusing to you. But if your child is truly shy, then what you perceive as indifference is likely to be a cover-up for the fear of rejection.

The self-talk of children is simpler than that of adults. Adults string together a series of possible scenarios in their automatic thoughts, recognizing that there are many ways people can respond. Children cannot think in gray areas and they do not consider exceptions to the rules. Their thinking tends to be concrete. This limits the variety of possible outcomes they can envision and can prevent them from assuming or even considering positive alternatives.

SHYNESS AND FEAR

Behind many shy behaviors lies anxiety, the most basic emotion we experience, the emotion welded to our survival mechanisms and least connected to our recently developed thinking brain. When we are confronted by something that scares us, our bodies react by freezing for an instant and then either confronting the source of the fear (fight) or running away from it (flight). However, one person's fear is another person's excitement. There are brave firefighters who will never set foot in an airplane because the thought of flying is too scary for them. Anxiety is the stronger emotion we experience and it is highly subjective.

Inordinate Self-consciousness

Many of the anxieties of shy children grow out of the fear of social evaluation. The shy child is hypersensitive to signals from other people indicating whether she is acting appropriately or if she is acceptable. Unfortunately, her negative self-talk and intensive perception of social situations make the shy child a bad judge of what other people truly feel about her. (See "Perceiving Reality," p. 42.) She may think she has been rejected, or that others are staring at her when, in fact, she is not being observed at all. Some shy children, for example, find it extremely difficult to eat in front of other people.

When you see your child hanging back on the playground, avoiding a conversation, or painfully preparing for a presentation, remember that he is nervous, unsure, and afraid. He is *frightened*—hold on to that thought without judging the source of his fear. This can be hard. It does not matter if you think it is silly to be afraid of a birthday party; your opinion of the fear will not reduce it. By belittling the fear, you can make the problem bigger by introducing more negative self-talk messages into your child's collection. "I shouldn't be afraid" is not a thought that really diminishes fear. It only adds to a sense of helplessness and self-doubt.

If you had been involved in a serious car crash, the sound of squealing brakes would likely make you nervous, causing you to relive your terror. Nobody would dream of telling you that your reaction was silly; they would sympathize and seek to calm your fears. In time, as you learned that not all squealing brakes guaranteed you two painful weeks in the hospital, your reactions would most likely diminish. That is the goal for your child—to slowly desensitize himself to the strong feelings that social situations create for him and to turn his pessimistic self-talk messages into neutral or positive ones.

A Confusing Ambivalence

The ambivalence of shy children can drive their parents to distraction. When Brittany sobs to her mother, "They're not paying any attention to me," her mother sympathizes, "It feels bad when people leave you out, doesn't it?" Brittany wipes her eyes on her sleeve, "Yes, but I hate it more when they notice me." Garrison Keillor, radio show host, comedian, author, and self-acknowledged shy person, said of his childhood, "I never wanted to be noticed at all, and at the same time I wanted people to bow down and worship me as the Sun God."

Shy children are, above all else, kids. They want to play with others. They want to have friends, to be at the center of a large adoring circle. They want to move with the ease and confidence they see in others; they want a friend to sit with at lunch; they want someone who will listen to their secrets. It would be easy to be shy if it weren't for these pesky, normal socialization desires.

Parents and children whipsaw back and forth between the emotional poles of desire and fear as the child wants to have friends, but reacts fearfully when socialization opportunities arise. The normal need for a friend is one of the best tools parents have. It is a wonderful carrot, a reward that will enrich your child for his entire life. The human craving to connect with other people can provide a wonderful balance to a shy child's fears.

Paralyzing Fear Versus Useful Anxiety

We automatically regard anxiety as a bad thing, but it isn't. Anxiety can prepare us for success. It can also be debilitating. An individual's reaction to anxiety depends on how she perceives the situation and how much control she thinks she has over her emotions.

Figure skater Michelle Kwan provided us with a marvelous example of the positive use of anxiety during the 1998 Olympics. Michelle skated disastrously during her warm-up for the short program—falling and faltering. She came off the ice, spoke briefly with her coach, then composed herself. The anxiety that tripped her up in the warm-up was channeled into focus and energy. She skated a tremendous short program, nearly flawless.

Anxiety is an internal barometer. We can acquaint our children with the sensations of anxiety, and the concept that anxiety in and of itself does not have to be a bad thing. Shy children feel so different from their peers that they may not believe that other kids have the same feelings or that mom or

dad feel anxious in some situations. Sharing your own moments of discomfort in a relaxed, open manner will help your
shy child view anxiety as a normal sensation, and learn to distinguish between degrees of anxiety. They can learn to identify the physical symptoms and to be alert to their self-talk
messages which exacerbate their anxiety. We must allow our
children to be comfortable with preparatory anxiety, to anticipate it, and to use it.

HOW A SHY CHILD SEES THE WORLD

Parents of shy children will immediately recognize that the
most difficult part of helping children to overcome fear is getting them to interpret a situation realistically. Shy children
often distort reality, and the distortion, which you can't always see, causes what may seem to you unreasonable fear. *You*
may assume that other children would be happy to have your
son sit with them at lunch, but he is convinced they will tell
him to get lost, or worse. How can he hope to develop social
skills when he can't even recognize the level of friendliness in
a cafeteria?

Perceiving Reality

Children typically go through two separate steps when they
enter an unfamiliar place. Their first move is called a "primary
appraisal" as they scan the room looking for reassurance or for
danger. When entering a new place, children look first for
things at their eye level; then they look up to assess which
adults are in the area.

   If a shy child judges the room to be safe for her, she can
relax and take in more information about her surroundings—

interesting books or toys, relaxing music, a trusted friend. If she finds something in her primary appraisal that alarms her, such as a loud group of boys, a stranger beckoning to her, or the immediate sense that there is no one familiar to her there, she will not gather more information. She will focus on what triggered the fear response in her. In doing so, she might distort both the scene that caught her attention and all the other information contained in the room.

While the child is seeking possible dangers, she is also evaluating her possible responses to a perceived threat. Can she walk out of the room? Cling to her mother? What will happen if she sits in the corner and doesn't say a word? This assessment of possible responses is called a "secondary appraisal."

It is not an exaggeration to say that a shy child entering a birthday party filled with unfamiliar children, blaring horns, balloons, and a large, red-nosed clown can have the same feelings an adult might have if dropped in a tiger's cage. Of course to you, this idea represents a distortion. But just imagine for a moment how it would feel if you thought you were in a tiger's cage. You are not going to observe the interesting species of orchid planted by the water bowl. You will remain fixated on the threat, not even noticing, perhaps, that the tiger is chained. Your self-talk would be filled with appraisals of how you can get out of there alive. If anyone dared to tell you that you are "being silly, it's just a big kitty-cat," your reaction would be less than polite. If others accused you of overreacting, you might be furious, or you might experience a moment of self-doubt. These are the emotions a shy child might feel whose parents insist she's overreacting by not joining the others at the birthday party.

It is shortsighted and harmful for us to expect our children to see the world the same way that we do. Perceptions are based on experience and the experiences of our children are necessarily quite different from ours. If you try to force your child to act the way you think she *should* in a given situation, she will dig in her heels and the problem will become worse. Your lack of understanding will strengthen her impression that something is wrong with her. If, on the other hand, you can accept that your child really does perceive things differently, then you can be more respectful and patient as you try to see the world through her lens. From this position of tolerance and respect, you can begin to help her put her world into perspective.

Perceiving Places

Shy children thrive in their comfort zones. Some children have extended zones that include their neighborhood, a few friends' homes, and school, while others have a smaller set of familiar places, their own house, perhaps the backyard. Within the comfort zone, a shy child is in control and not afraid to show all the parts of her personality, but stick her in an unfamiliar setting, and she pulls into her shell. Author and philosopher Franz Kafka described this feeling in a letter.

> But if I am in an unfamiliar place, among a number of strange people, or people whom I feel to be strangers, then the whole room presses on my chest and I am unable to move, my whole personality seems virtually to get under their skins, and everything becomes hopeless.—June 1913
>
> [quoted in *Solitude: A Return to the Self*, Anthony Storr, p. 101]

Your child's bedroom may be the center of her comfort zone. Some shy children hate redecorating their room or throwing out old toys, books, or bedspreads because every item is part of what makes the room so familiar. The rest of the house will likely be included in the comfort zone, though adjusting after a move can take longer for shy children.

Your child's level of ease in your neighborhood will be influenced by how friendly she is with the other people she sees when she plays outside. If she is constantly assessing how she will be received by other children, or if adults mowing their lawns or washing cars talk to her and make her self-conscious, then she will probably spend more time inside.

School can be both a familiar and unfamiliar place. If your child's school is large, and the makeup of classes changes annually, then your child can be back at square one every September, forced to cope with the anxieties evoked by a new classroom, teacher, and classmates, as well as rising academic and social expectations. It's the tiger's cage all over again. Even within a comfortable classroom setting, specific school activities can trigger shy behavior and anxiety in your child. For a shy child, celebrations such as Valentine's Day can be excruciating and anticipating oral reports can ruin a whole week.

Watch how your child acts the next time you take her to a familiar place like the grocery store, mall, or library. If it is part of your normal routine, she will be relaxed and playful. If you visit a new place, she may act up or withdraw. Your child might throw a temper tantrum out of her sense of being overwhelmed, or will make the excursion as miserable as possible to cut it short. You may feel manipulated and frustrated by this behavior; rightly so. However, as we will discuss at length later, the time to deal with these confrontations is not in the middle of the store. Patience and planning ahead pay off. As you work through the exercises described later in the book, your shy child will develop a tolerance for new settings, and you will know how to plan for introducing them to her. As your child learns to feel more self-confident, she will enjoy the positive, exciting aspects of visiting new places, and she will know how to cope with any anxiety that unfamiliar places may touch off.

What are your child's comfort zones? Where does her personality bubble out and where does she clam up, observing intently and keeping to herself? Watch your child for the next week and note where she feels safe enough to be herself.

MY CHILD'S COMFORT ZONE

Places where my child is completely comfortable:

_____

Possible reasons based on his perceptions:

_____

Places where my child is slightly anxious:

_____

Possible reasons based on his perceptions:

_____

Places where my child is uncomfortable:

_____

Possible reasons based on his perceptions:

_____

Places where my child hates to go:

_____

Possible reasons based on his perceptions:

_____

Perceiving People

Since shyness is a set of anxieties arising from social interactions, dealing with people is the single most difficult task a shy child must confront. But once a shy child becomes comfortable with a new person, once he trusts that the person accepts him without judgment and enjoys spending time with him, the barriers fall. The challenge for parents is to understand how a new person affects their child.

Shy children do not see other kids as automatic playmates. A new child may appear as a threat, someone to avoid. The first response of a shy child may be, "What does she want from me?" or "What am I supposed to do?" instead of assuming the new child is a nice person who wants to play. The physical behaviors of a shy child—turning his head to avoid the other child's eyes, refusing to speak, or freezing—will not elicit friendly feedback from a new child. The shy child may be thought to be indifferent or stuck up—not a good way to begin a friendship.

Relatives can seem just as hostile and scary as complete strangers. Your child may not warm up to grandparents that he only sees once a year if there is no continuation of contact between visits. Just because you say grandma and grandpa love him doesn't mean he can drop all his defenses and throw himself at people to whom he does not feel connected. Some shy children have a hard time talking on the telephone, so do not assume that phone calls to distant relatives will pave the way to a relationship when they visit. If the phone stresses your child, he may barely remember the conversation after he hangs up.

Imagine yourself walking down a dangerous street as the sun is setting. Sure, intellectually you know that the chances of something bad happening are slim. But is that man staring at you? Those kids over there, they're acting suspicious. Should you run? Are you going to get out of this in one piece? That's the level of tension a shy child can experience around strangers, even as a well-meaning parent or teacher is telling him to relax and smile.

As you try to see the world with your shy child's eyes, remember that he thinks in stark, black-and-white terms; there is no middle ground, no compromise, no gray. A situation is comfortable or uncomfortable; a person is safe or scary. As you work with your child to identify his self-talk and show him how to control his anxiety level and acclimate to the sensations of socialization, his world will widen and he will grow more confident of his place in it.

Watch your child in public settings for the next few days. Carefully observe his body language for signs of anxiety and stress, particularly as he interacts with others. Who is inside your child's circle of trust and who stands on the fringes?

MY CHILD'S CIRCLE OF TRUST

Who makes my child totally at ease?

_____

Possible reasons based on her perceptions:

_____

Who makes my child slightly anxious?

_____

Possible reasons based on her perceptions:

_____

Who makes my child uncomfortable?

_____

Possible reasons based on her perceptions:

_____

Who makes my child frightened?

_____

Possible reasons based on her perceptions:

_____

Overwhelmed and Overstimulated

Matthew was a beautiful, moon-faced baby with serious chocolate brown eyes that followed his mother's every move. As a baby, he had a definite comfort zone; he could not stand for strangers to get too close to him. If anyone crossed Matthew's boundary, he would bare his teeth at them and growl like a wild animal. This behavior shocked and embarrassed his outgoing mother. She was extremely social and wanted her baby to join play groups and feel as comfortable with others as she did. "It was very hard to deal with," she says. "He wasn't like me."

Things came to a head with Matthew during a birthday party at a play center, attended by all his preschool classmates. While the other boys were becoming more and more hyperactive and loud—thanks to the music, the video games, and the swirl of activity—Matthew stayed close to his mother and periodically begged to go home. She blithely told him no, because this was fun, and why didn't he go and try out the area where all the kids were frolicking knee-deep in plastic balls. She wasn't noticing his increasing distress, because he was very quiet and observant. Finally, he began to cry, and when a teacher noticed, he became embarrassed; his face turned beet red, and he screamed in anger until his mother led him away.

"I was mortified," she remembers. "What did I do wrong? I thought he was just being stubborn, and then, when he made a scene, I thought he was trying to manipulate me into taking him home."

Many shy people perceive the world as an extremely intense place. Shy adults report that they are easily overstimulated by such things as fluorescent lights, rooms with more than one conversation going on, the sensation of being crowded in a subway. These adults sometimes feel an inability to filter out sensory awareness. They absorb details of every person in a crowd: their clothes, attitudes, their perfume. They are hypersensitive to their surroundings.

It is suspected that shy children experience the same sensations, though they cannot describe them. Indeed, they probably don't realize that not everyone feels the same way.

While some children react to overstimulation by getting louder, faster, and more and more out of control, the shy child may have a completely different reaction. Children tend to act out their emotions. He might wander away from a group to sit alone. He may retreat into a bathroom and lock the door or "zone out" in front of the television or a video game.

After a trip to the mall, your shy child might seem completely wrung out. She might be very quiet and express a desire just to go to her room and be alone. She needs that time to regain her equilibrium. If prevented for some reason, or if the overstimulation continues, she may grow quieter and quieter until finally erupting in rage. The intensity of a shy child's tantrums can be all the more surprising because it seems so uncharacteristic for "the quiet one."

When a child as young as Matthew reaches his snapping point, he has nowhere to go with his emotions but out. It took his mother several years to understand that her son did not enjoy the social outings she took him on, but that he was a wonderful, loving child who noticed butterflies and loved trains. Matthew has grown into a sensitive, confident young man because his mother recognized what triggered anxiety in him and helped him take control in different situations. Children who do not learn to master the overwhelming feelings of isolation in overstimulating environments can turn their anger inward and become depressed.

A NOTE ON DEPRESSION

A shy child can appear to be a depressed child, and children who are depressed often exhibit shy behaviors, but shyness and depression are two separate problems. It is not the case that shyness is a mild version of depression, nor is there evidence that childhood depression is the end result of untreated shyness. However, shy children can slip into depression like any other children, and parents must be vigilant.

Depression can show up in children as young as four years old. According to the American Psychiatric Association, as many as one in ten children aged six to twelve suffer from depression. Some of the symptoms of depression appear to be shyness behaviors on the surface, such as withdrawal or heightened levels of anxiety. But a depressed child will display a spirit of hopelessness: he gives up on the world, and sees no way out of his storm of negative feelings. Parents need to be aware of the behavioral changes that signal depression. Watch for increased irritability, aggression, changes in eating or sleeping patterns, giving away possessions, a sense of hopelessness, a sudden drop in school performance, antisocial behavior, sadness, and the use of alcohol or other drugs.

A shy child can become a depressed child. This can happen anytime, but parents should pay special attention during adolescence, when all children develop a heightened awareness of the opinion of their peers and experience more self-doubt. Shy teenagers tend to set extremely high, sometimes unrealistic, goals for themselves, such as perfect SAT scores or admission into an Ivy League university. Falling short of these goals can reinforce negative self-talk messages and begin a downward spiral into despair. Shy children can also become depressed if there are conflicts within their family such as divorce or a move and if they are not given the necessary attention and opportunities to air feelings and fears.

Depression in children is a serious issue. Children who feel hopeless and see no way out of their pain may hurt themselves, either with self-destructive behaviors or by committing suicide. It does not matter if the depression is rooted in brain chemistry or problems the child is facing; the feelings and consequences are the same. If you suspect your child is depressed in addition to being shy, you should seek professional help. Please contact your pediatrician or family physician immediately.

INTROVERSION VERSUS EXTROVERSION

Most people, if asked, will describe introverts as quiet persons who prefer solitude over the company of others and introspection over activity. Introverts seem inhibited; they need a lot of time alone to rebalance their energies. Extroverts are the opposite of introverts. They not only enjoy, but crave the company of others. They are active, gregarious, and bold. It can be said that introverts shy away from the outside world and extroverts shy away from the inside world.

The concept of introvert and extrovert came out of the work of pioneering psychologist Carl Jung. Jung described the relationship between introverted and extroverted qualities as a kind of teeter-totter. Contrary to popular belief, no one is purely an introvert or purely an extrovert; we each have some of each quality. Most shy children, however, clearly exhibit more introverted traits.

The Interior Life of the Introvert

Our culture does not champion introverts. People who want to spend time alone are suspect; they are thought to be hiding something; they are odd. We pity the person eating alone in a restaurant, and we wonder about the child who prefers to go off by himself. We expect everyone to join in group activities and participate enthusiastically. Other cultures are more forgiving of the need for solitude and allow for time and space to be set aside for those who need to recharge their psychic batteries in solitude. Some other cultures, it must be said, are even less understanding of introversion than our own.

The American preference for extroversion blinds us to the wonderful features of the introvert's personality. Introverts are thoughtful and sensitive. They usually empathize well with others. Introverts have contributed enormously to music, literature, and the visual arts. Their ability to remain focused for long periods of time while alone makes them successful as researchers and theoretical mathematicians. For the same reason that they are easily overstimulated, introverts have an eye for detail and an ear for nuance. They are constantly responding to internal stimuli—some say they have "tapes" continually running in their heads that allow them to synthesize information in interesting ways.

They may not be surrounded by a pack of friends like extroverts are, but they are fiercely loyal and supportive of the friends they have. It can take longer to get to know an introvert, but the effort pays off handsomely when you discover what treasures are hiding beneath the quiet surface.

In the negative column, however, introverts are likely to shut themselves off from new experiences. They sometimes need a gentle push to explore territory beyond what is familiar and comfortable. They are not good at self-promotion, and consequently they might hide their lights under the proverbial bushel basket. Competition, another quality admired in American culture, can make them uncomfortable.

Shy Extroverts

Corbin is a gifted soccer player. The nine-year-old has amazing coordination and speed, combined with a love of the sport. He is also a good organizer and leader. The other boys on his team recognize his gifts and are very happy to have him on the team. When Corbin scores a goal, they gather round him and cheer. But Corbin has no friends.

When he is off the soccer field, he is unsure how to relate to the other boys. He doesn't know how to talk to them, what to say. He lacks the ability to connect with them. He plays best in a highly structured situation such as a soccer match. Corbin's talents make him appear to be outgoing, but he must learn how to develop friendships. He is a shy extrovert.

A shy extrovert is not an oxymoron. In fact, many shy children grow up and become shy extroverts, though they usually are described differently. Shy extroverts have mastered the structure of specific social situations. They can "perform" without anxiety, but don't know how to relate to their peers in personal relationships. There are many adults who feel as if they have outgrown their childhood shyness, but who are really shy extroverts. They have learned to manage their shyness in the workplace, for example, but they feel lonely, even if they have friends and a spouse.

These adults did not learn how to connect with other people when they were children. Back then, their social awkwardness isolated them and caused tremendous pain. They built walls to protect themselves from the pain of social interactions; they learned to act indifferent instead of afraid when confronting new people or new situations. In their adult life, they may feel empty and confused and may not make the connection to their childhood shyness. A shy extrovert is like an actor who cries behind his mask.

The terms *introvert* and *extrovert* can be useful in understanding what makes your child tick. But your shy child is a blend of both introverted and extroverted characteristics. You may see that blend shift as your child matures and her response to life experiences pushes her further inward or draws her out into more of a social person. Wherever your child falls on the introversion–extroversion spectrum, be alert to her unique, positive traits, and look for ways that she can be supported and embraced for the kind of person she is.

USING COGNITIVE THERAPY TO TREAT SHYNESS IN CHILDREN

Our approach to assessing and "treating" shyness in *The Sky Child* comes out of cognitive therapy, an approach to working out anxiety issues that contains elements of behavioral and cognitive theories. Cognitive therapy (sometimes called cognitive-behavioral therapy) is based on the concept that thoughts directly influence our emotions. When people are taught how to examine their thoughts (hear their self-talk), realistically evaluate the things that make them anxious, and develop a sense of control and mastery over their emotions, they can reduce their anxiety and perform unhampered in life.

Martin E. P. Seligman, Ph.D., psychology professor at the University of Pennsylvania, designed the Penn Prevention Program to help fifth- and sixth-grade children who were at risk for depression develop techniques that would prevent depression from overwhelming their lives. Part of the program involved training the children to examine their automatic thoughts and take control of them, with the hope that eliminating negative self-talk and improving social skills would make the children happier.

Seligman and his team worked with seventy children for a year, then followed the students for two more years to measure the long-term impact of the training. Immediately after the program ended, there was a 35 percent reduction in the number of children showing strong depressive symptoms. Two years later, this number increased to 100 percent; impressive results indeed. These numbers are even more dramatic in light of the fact that the targeted children were going through adolescence during the period of the study, which Seligman thought would increase the number of students who would become depressed. Children in the control group, who had not been trained in the techniques of self-talk mastery and social interaction skills, showed a much greater increase in depressive symptoms.

Dr. Aaron Beck is a professor of psychiatry at the University of Pennsylvania School of Medicine and director of the Center of Cognitive Thought in Philadelphia. Along with his colleagues, he has been exploring the connections between our thoughts and our emotions for the past thirty years. With its effectiveness proven by countless studies, cognitive therapy is now recognized as an extremely useful form of therapy for many disorders.

Patients who work with psychological professionals using a cognitive therapy approach spend a relatively short time in therapy, generally no more than a few months. They are given homework assignments and learn many tools they continue to use after the therapy is complete. These tools work very well within the context of a family, and the cognitive therapy model is well suited to adaptation for use by parents with shy children.

Using the cognitive therapy model, you will help your child:

- Identify negative self-talk;
- Modify negative self-talk to neutral or positive messages;
- Find connections between self-talk and emotional responses;
- Perceive social situations accurately;
- Practice social interactive tasks in safe settings;
- Develop repetitive behaviors for stressful situations; and
- Review failure, restructure new plans, and celebrate success.

CHAPTER SUMMARY

1. Understanding what goes on in the mind of a shy child can help a parent empathize and guide with wisdom.

2. Self-talk is the constant flow of automatic thoughts that go on in the mind.

3. Self-talk can be positive or negative.

4. Shy children experience a heightened degree of critical self-talk which gnaws at their confidence and inhibits their behavior.

5. Shy children are hyper-responsive in social situations. They tend to perceive social situations poorly.

6. Shy children are easily overstimulated, which further provokes feelings of being out of place.

7. Shyness is driven by anxiety and fear.

8. Most shy children show introverted characteristics, but some can appear extroverted.

9. Shyness can lead to depression when a child's feelings of exclusion or low self-worth run out of control.

10. Cognitive therapy provides parents with effective tools for helping their shy children reduce anxiety levels.

Chapter 3

HOW DID THIS HAPPEN?

Parents often subject themselves to deep feelings of self-doubt when it comes to their children's developing personalities and behaviors. A mother whose small son begins to suck his thumb regrets that she stopped breast-feeding him and blames herself. A father whose daughter has temper tantrums well into her teens suspects that his own volatility provided a poor example of how to handle anger. A child who cries easily has parents who fear they have not taught him to be tough. And the parents of a petulant child who always demands her own way fear they have spoiled her. Inevitably parents do influence their child's behavior. But it is far too simple to assume that the decisions parents make are the only influences on their children.

Thirty years ago experts felt that children were born with a more or less clean slate, and that their personalities developed as a result of their experiences and the type of world they lived in. Experts in the field of genetics are working toward tipping the nature versus nurture argument back in favor of nature. There is evidence that who we are in terms of basic personality style is also influenced by our genetic makeup. However, this news does not let parents off the hook altogether. If, as the evidence suggests, we are *born* with a good deal of our temperament, that temperament must be viewed in combination with our life experiences to explain how we end up with our complete, adult personalities.

Quite naturally, the parents of shy children—those who feel that the extent of the shyness is inhibiting their child's happiness—wonder if something about their way of interacting has caused this personality style to develop. It is not out of the question, as we shall see, that parenting styles and external events can lead outgoing children to become more withdrawn. But if that is so, then it is also true that parenting styles can lead introverted children to become more comfortable with their world, which is, of course, the subject of this book. As the information in this chapter implies, shyness is a natural personality style that can be influenced by both nature *and* nurture. Understanding how both impact on your child's personality development can help you embrace her shyness as well as assist her in keeping it from slowing her down.

BORN SHY?

It was hard to find Emily in photographs. The tiny young woman always stood behind the crowd or turned away from the camera at the right moment. Intensely shy, she only felt comfortable with close family members and a few friends known since she was a baby.

Pictures were important to Emily's family. She had inherited artistic talent from her father, a college English professor who painted beautiful landscapes in his spare time. Emily was born with the same ability, though her desire to become a better artist was frustrated by her shyness. She hated starting a new art class; having to introduce herself; not knowing what to say to the other students; wanting the teacher to read her mind and know the kind of help she needed.

Emily thought something was seriously wrong with her, something that set her apart from everyone else she knew. No one else seemed to agonize the way she did. Wherever she looked, she saw relaxed, happy art students, eagerly comparing techniques and secrets. Her confusion and anxiety built until she couldn't stand the art classes anymore, even though painting was one of the few ways she could express herself. She stopped going to class.

Emily's mother was the complete opposite of her daughter. She was outgoing, forthright, determined, and active. Her daughter's reticence worried her, though her quiet, gentle husband counseled patience. He knew that Emily had to find her own way. Her mother convinced Emily to help her with genealogy research. Spending hours in silent libraries surrounded by dusty books was more comfortable than having to think of something to say to fellow art students, and Emily agreed.

Mother and daughter found much more than an impressive family tree. They interviewed relatives and uncovered strong family characteristics that had been

passed on from generation to generation. The
mother's inexhaustible energy and drive came from
Scottish immigrants. Emily's younger sister's piano
talents could be traced back to a Civil War bugler.
Emily herself was one of the "quiet ones," relatives
and ancestors who kept to the sidelines, but who were
enormously perceptive and sensitive. She wasn't weird
or crazy; she just came from a long line of shy people.

Seeing herself as one member of a group of shy
people comforted Emily. It gave her a sense of belonging and helped ease her anxiety. Her mother
made sure that Emily did not use this new knowledge
as an excuse to avoid new situations. Instead, armed
with the understanding that shyness was a core part of
her personality, Emily was able to approach new situations more confidently.

Science is beginning to agree with anecdotal evidence,
such as stories of the shy branches on Emily's family tree,
which implies that shyness is a characteristic that can be
handed down from generation to generation much the same
way that red hair or dimples are. In fact, parents can receive
clues about their baby's temperament before the child is born.
Some babies are "kickers" in the womb, while others are
"floaters." Once the child is born, his parents must discover
what level of stimulation he likes and how he prefers to relate
to the world.

Studies in Shyness

Jerome Kagan, a pioneering developmental psychologist at
Harvard University, has studied hundreds of children and de-

termined that some shyness is "hardwired." That is to say that some children are born with inhibited tendencies that make them freeze in unfamiliar situations, keep quiet around strangers, avoid new stimulus, and withdraw into themselves when stressed.

Kagan and his team monitored the reactions of four-month-old babies to colorful mobiles, voices, and smells. Infants who reacted by crying, arching their backs, and moving their arms and legs violently were categorized as highly reactive. The infants who watched placidly or with interest without showing signs of distress were classified as low reactive. There were two intermediate categories: one for children whose reactions were classified as distressed, and the other, which was classified as aroused.

Kagan followed up with these children at fourteen and twenty-one months, and again when the children were three and a half years old. He found that those children who were most distressed by sights, sounds, and smells during the first test grew into children who exhibited a number of shy behaviors. In later tests, they were likely to turn away from a stranger walking into a room, to run back to their mother for comfort, to freeze or refuse to speak, and to show uncertainty and discomfort in unfamiliar surroundings. Babies who had remained relaxed or even interested during the earlier trials grew up into children who openly greeted strangers, talked to new children easily, were eager for new experiences, and could laugh at their mistakes.

Based on years of detailed research and analysis, Kagan concluded that 20 percent of children are born with a shy or inhibited temperament. He believes that the brains of these children are more easily aroused to anticipate fear and danger when other children do not sense any trouble. At the other end of the scale, Kagan found 40 percent of children to be born with relaxed, easygoing personalities that do not react with fear or anxiety to new situations. If these two groups are understood to be poles of introversion (inhibited) and extroversion (uninhibited), then the remaining 40 percent of children fall somewhere in the middle.

HONORING YOUR CHILD'S STYLE

Will scientists ever be able to pinpoint the genes that determine shy tendencies? Focusing on that quest does not help us. Children come into the world with a partially written script. Environment, parenting, and opportunity will always have important influences on the kind of people they become. The path to success in parenting children of any temperament is to strive to understand the kind of temperament your child was born with by noticing what kind of activity makes him happy; how he likes to play; what soothes him; what disturbs him. Knowing all of this is one thing, but respecting and honoring your child's style of interacting with the world is the key to making sure his temperament does not trip him up later in life.

It helps parents to be aware how their children are influenced by the daily events of life and by the more serious complications that can intrude into childhood. Every child's personality is a blend of inborn characteristics and experience. By understanding a child's inborn temperament and recognizing the influence of daily events, we can best nurture him to enjoy the fullest quality of life.

MADE SHY? THE ROLE OF EXPERIENCE

What about those children who are not born with shy tendencies? What can turn an outgoing child into an inhibited one? Just as not all the inhibited babies in Kagan's study grew into shy children, some of the fearless babies developed into bashful toddlers. Kagan found that the way parents interact with their children does affect personality, either validating and thus intensifying the natural, genetic tendency toward introversion or extroversion, or ameliorating those traits, thus making the naturally shy child more outgoing or the naturally nonshy child more reticent.

It is clear that environment has a critical influence. Shyness is determined both by nature and nurture, or as Christine Hohmann, a neuroscientist at the Kennedy-Kriger Institute in Baltimore, put it in a *Los Angeles Times* article: "The genes are the bricks and mortar to build a brain. The environment is the architect."

Social Factors

Pressures from school, among friends, or in the family can turn an uninhibited child into a withdrawn one. Parents need to understand how different types of social factors affect their children's perception of themselves and how that self-perception, if negative, can eat away at children's confidence and limit their happiness. Children exhibit shy tendencies when they are feeling anxious. When the world threatens to overwhelm them, they pull into themselves. If relating to others becomes painful, they stop, and this behavior, when reinforced, can develop into shyness. They require a higher level of comfort and security at times like these. It is important not to judge your child's needs ("Don't be ridiculous; all the other children are singing on the stage") but instead to examine the situation, understand what is fueling your child's anxiety, and work together to increase her confidence and comfort in order to work through the anxiety.

Events in a child's life that parents may not define as traumatic can take on traumatic proportions in a child's worldview and lead to a temporary change in behavior.

Brian's parents had never considered him shy; he was more outgoing than his older brother and was a normally confident, sometimes boisterous, little boy. He was an excellent piano player and an average student with plenty of friends both in his neighborhood and at school. But toward the end of fourth grade, Brian underwent a major personality change that seemed to occur overnight. He withdrew from playing outside, refusing to come to the phone or answer the door when his friends called. He stopped playing the piano—a complete shock, as he had never had to be reminded to practice before. He followed his parents constantly, unable even to be on a different floor of the house from them. "It seemed like he went into a cocoon," his father said.

Brian's parents took him to a child psychologist. Brian was slightly anxious about his schoolwork, but he was extremely upset about a problem between two sets of friends. Both group of boys wanted Brian to hang out with them and were pressuring him to abandon the other group. Brian felt torn and confused; he couldn't even articulate his emotions or describe what was going on to his parents.

Brian's inability to put his emotions into words was very important. He honestly could not share what he was feeling, and didn't have a hope of sorting it out on his own. The hostile pressure he was getting from two groups of boys made him overly sensitive to what others thought of him and made all kinds of social situations unpleasant. With strong emotions rocketing through him, he responded by withdrawing because he found it easier to stay safe in his house than to deal with the difficult and confusing conflict.

His parents were horrified at first because they felt they had failed—they had not been aware of the problems with Brian's friends and they had no idea how upset he was. They were filled with doubts about themselves—how could they have missed this? The psychologist pointed out that they had done everything right. They hadn't overreacted when Brian began to withdraw, they tried to get him to talk about what was bothering him, and when they had reached the limit of their skills, they brought in a professional. Parents cannot monitor children twenty-four hours a day. Even if they could, that would not be healthy. Children must learn to cope with the unfamiliar and the difficult; in fact, it is better for them to come up against difficult social situations when they are young and under the care of their parents so that they have love and support to help them work through their problems.

After the situation was identified and Brian learned

how to cope with the pressures of the friends, he regained his self-confidence. He returned to his piano playing and took up the drums. His father feels he came out of his cocoon a stronger boy than when he went in: "He just needed to figure out how to deal with it all. Now he's happy."

Response to Trauma

Genuine trauma also moderates the inborn temperament of children, and a percentage of children develop withdrawal in response to an early traumatic experience. Trauma can be defined as normal—that is, the uncertainty that accompanies milestones in life that all people experience—or serious, involving a death in the family, catastrophic illness or injury, divorce, or abuse. The severity of the experience, the age when it occurred, and the family response to the event all affect how withdrawn the child becomes. There is also the indefinable nature of the child's character. Some children seem to be born more resilient than others and will come through difficult emotional trauma less affected.

Normal Trauma. Normal traumas are the heart-wrenching experiences of childhood. Everybody has to muddle through normal trauma as best we can. Children who are naturally self-assured usually come through normal trauma relatively unscathed, but some find that a series of upsets can cause personality changes, making them withdraw from activities they once enjoyed and becoming anxious and doubtful. Shy children can be deeply injured by trauma.

Developmental Milestones. Children are apt to feel more anxious as they pass through their physical and emotional developmental milestones, such as crawling, walking, and separating from parents. Just as a child can be unexplainedly cranky for a few days before a new tooth pops out, the interior stresses of growing up can make a child fretful. Chapters 5 through 10 will take you step by step through the developmental stages of childhood and help explain why your child responds the way he does and how you can help him feel more comfortable. Below are some general milestones that tend to lead shy children to become more withdrawn and outgoing children to behave more like shy children.

New Baby. A new baby in the house stresses everyone, but no one more than the older sibling who may not even have the words to explain his feelings. Most parents expect their older child to need more attention and tender, loving care when a new baby comes home, but few expect a personality change.

School. School is the central social experience for most children. While school is in session, your child will spend more than half of his waking hours traveling to or from school, in the classroom, or working on homework. As Brian's parents found out, social conflicts that take place in school can be difficult to discover because many children are reluctant to talk about school problems.

Going to school is filled with vulnerable moments that can make a child who is not temperamentally inhibited into a child afraid to make social contact. Children can be overwhelmed by the combination of academic expectations and social pressures. A child who is not athletic will forever remember the pain of gym class, or of being chosen last for playground sports. Kids who don't form strong social circles learn to hate lunch; they suffer through that awkward moment coming out of the lunch line, they're not sure whom to sit with, and they have to watch "successful" friendships all around them.

Some children develop horrendous stress about making good grades. They internalize their parents' instructions to excel, and are constantly aware of their grades and of upcoming tests, reports, and projects. If these pressures build in a negative way, the child feels under a constant cloud. She worries about everything she does in class and dreads each assignment. In time, this anxiety can grow to the point where it actually interferes with her schoolwork.

Teasing. Children who feel vulnerable in school or social settings are at greater risk for being teased or bullied. They don't fight back, they won't confront their tormentor, and they rarely tell the adults around them what is going on. This is the perfect situation for the bully.

A shy child, or a child who is going through a period of shyness, can be scarred by a bully. The aggressive tormentor reinforces the negative self-talk already playing in the mind of the victim, telling him that he's different, that no one likes him, that he's useless, that he's weak. Children who have a strong social base or self-confidence can stand up to this kind of teasing or walk away from it. Anxious children can be wounded by it.

Moving. Moving is difficult for everyone at every age. It can have significant long-term impact on children. A child who was secure in his previous home may be completely thrown by a move. He may develop shy behavior for the first time. Children who are not temperamentally shy may act clingy in the new home or resentful at the loss of friends and familiar places. Most will adjust within a few months and enjoy their new home.

For some children, a move can disrupt their lives more seriously. Parents need to try to experience a move from their child's perspective. There is often tension in the house as a move is debated. There are the stresses of selling a home, and sometimes separation as one parent moves ahead to take a new job. The child watches as his world is packed into boxes and carted away. He is left with crushing feelings of sadness. He has no control over what is happening. At the time when he most needs comfort and attention, family members are distracted by the moving process. Finally, the family moves into the new house. Sometimes parents offer toys or the chance to paint their bedroom to make a child feel better. It is not enough.

For a shy child, moving can be a particularly trying time. Home is the one stable place a shy child has. It is his fortress, his retreat. Many shy children are reluctant even to redecorate their rooms, because the disruption is too hard for them. One boy protested every time his mother changed the sheets on his bed.

Moving can push a shy child toward severe anxiety on the shyness spectrum. Parents need to be aware of this and work with their child to help her deal with her feelings of anxiety and anger. Just as a child who develops shyness during a move can regain her former self-confidence, a shy child can eventually work her way back toward a more balanced, healthy perspective.

Poor Parenting. There is no question about it: poor parenting can make a child withdrawn, anxious, and shy. On the other hand, good parenting can help even the shyest child feel more confident of her place in the world. If a parent constantly shelters and protects a child and gives the impression that the world is a hostile, dangerous place, the child will learn that timid behavior is a good thing. Parents who show a child how to take appropriate risks such as walking, exploring, and meeting new children present the world as an exciting challenge, not a constant source of fear.

Profound Trauma. Children who live through the death of a family member or close friend, sexual molestation or physical abuse, or divorce can come through the experience with radical personality changes. Profound traumas like these can forever shut away an outgoing, effervescent child. Parents must recognize the long-term impact that serious trauma can have on a child; a situation compounded by the fact that traumas such as these tend to impact an entire family, and parents may be having a hard time holding themselves together. Serious trauma does not mean that a child is sentenced to a life of misery, but is a signal that a child will need a great deal of support and understanding.

Death. When a parent dies, the surviving spouse can be so overwhelmed that behavioral changes in a child go unnoticed, or the parent does not have the emotional resources to respond to them. Other family members or friends may need to step in to make sure that a child's needs are met.

Alissa was a shy first grader, but she had friends and participated in class. At the beginning of second grade, she acted like a different child. Alissa did not say anything, not a single word to anyone. She was withdrawn and refused to do anything in the classroom. Her teacher contacted Alissa's mother to discuss the situation and quickly learned the root of the problem. Alissa's father had been killed over the summer. Alissa's mother did not allow her to talk about the father's death at all, not even at home. The teacher helped the family find the help they needed. It took some time, but Alissa slowly came to terms with her father's death and emerged as a confident happy child again.

Children are also deeply affected when their friends die. Parents must ensure their children have plenty of opportunities to talk about their feelings and slowly come to terms with the loss. Many schools offer counseling when a student dies. If the friend of a shy child dies, the negative impact can be even greater. Shy children do not develop many close friendships. They tend to be selective, cautious, and loyal. Parents should consider seeking professional assistance to help their child cope with the loss.

Molestation and Abuse. Sexual molestation of a child ranks high on the list of parental nightmares. Shy children may be less at risk for molestation by strangers because they are more cautious and would be less inclined to talk to strangers. Unfortunately most child sexual molestations are committed by people that the child knows well. Children are often threatened with punishment by molesters if they tell of the abuse. This type of fear is exacerbated by the shy child's harsh self-view.

Parents should take action if their child suddenly makes a radical change in behavior that cannot be explained by an obvious traumatic event. Molestation can turn a quiet child into a silent child. He may experience nightmares. He may be afraid to leave the house. Teachers may report behavioral changes in school.

A child who was not born shy can develop shyness as a result of molestation. The horror of molestation can replay in the mind of a child, making him view himself with loathing and contempt. He may grow oversensitive to what others think of him. He may long to play with friends, but feel afraid to relate to others. The family of a molestation victim needs to work with professionals to help the child regain a sense of trust in the world and restore his shaken self-confidence.

Divorce. Divorce is, sadly, the most common of the serious life traumas that can affect the basic temperament of children. Close to half of the children in America experience the breakup of their parents' marriage. Divorce can make children feel helpless, abandoned, even worthless or guilty if they think they caused the divorce. These feelings can be so overwhelming that a child might shut down. Unable to sort out her own emotions, she might pull away from all social contact.

Assessing Your Child's Shyness

Understanding the roots of your child's shyness will help you respond to his behaviors appropriately. In light of the above discussion on inborn or experience-driven shyness, write down your evaluation of your child's shy behaviors, where they might have come from, and what types of situations are most difficult.

Relatives who are shy:

Shy behaviors shown as a baby (see Chapter 5 for some examples):

Situations that make my child feel shy:

Situations in which my child feels and acts confidently:

Recent developmental milestones:

Possible serious traumas my child has experienced:

Issues that are difficult for my child to discuss:

HOW THE BRAIN WORKS

Just as science is uncovering that some people are born with a predisposition to shy behavior and others develop shyness in response to life events, we are learning that some shy behaviors are not conscious choices, but are physical reactions to stimuli. Research into the circuitry of the brain itself can help us understand what goes on deep in the brain of a child who is terrified of speaking in front of a class, and why he cannot get the words out. It also shows us how we can help that child take charge of his body's reactions and become comfortable in situations that once paralyzed him.

The brain differences of a temperamentally shy child and a child who has developed shy behaviors may simply be matters of degree. There is much work yet to be done in this field. But evidence of the chain of events that links certain stimuli to shy reactions is convincing.

Brain 101

To understand the brain, it helps to learn a few basics. The brain is the center of our thoughts, our emotions, and the control of our bodies. The relationships between these aspects is rich and complex. Parts of the brain work automatically; you breathe, your heart beats, and your eyes blink without any conscious thought on your part. Other activities require varying levels of effort and concentration, such as cocking your wrist at a different angle to make a basketball go through the net or analyzing a spreadsheet.

Different regions of the brain control different types of activity, although there have been cases of people whose injured brains have "rerouted" tasks to healthy regions. Three sections of the brain have come under the spotlight in the search for a biological root for anxiety: the thalamus, the neocortex, and the amygdala.

The thalamus is a gatekeeper of the brain. All sensory information, with the exception of smell, travels through the thalamus: The sound of a door slamming, the sight of a sunset over the desert, the taste of pumpkin pie, or the feeling of a splinter in your toe are first felt as nervous impulses in the thalamus, and then sent to the sensory-processing areas of the neocortex.

The neocortex is the largest part of our brain; it is where most of the "thinking," our cognitive functions and perceptual processes, takes place. Human beings are born with the structure of the neocortex in place and we spend our lifetime accumulating the memories and knowledge that are stored in and accessed by the neocortex. The neocortex allows us to anticipate and to act, to remember, to dream, and to create.

The third player in all behavior, including shy behavior, is the amygdala. The amygdala is a small, almond-shaped structure that nestles above the brainstem. It is a relatively "old" brain structure in that it is found in most mammals. The amygdala is considered one of the emotional centers of the brain; some call it the center of passion. It allows us to love and mourn, to celebrate and rage. Significantly, the activity of the amygdala is triggered by norepinephrine, a kind of adrenaline that floods the body in stressful situations.

Traditional scientific theory held that sensory signals were sent first to the thalamus and then to the neocortex, where the thinking brain processed them. Anything that required an emotional response was then routed to the amygdala, which knew what type of emotion was called for. When you held your child for the first time, it "accessed" joy. When a bully cornered you in the schoolyard, it triggered anger. When you headed into an automobile accident, it signaled fear. And so on.

New Research on the Role of the Amygdala and Its Significance in Shyness

Neurobiologists and psychologists have recently confirmed evidence that points to a different sequence of events. Joseph LeDoux, Ph.D., professor of psychology and neuroscience at New York University, has spent years investigating the mysteries of the amygdala. LeDoux started with rats whose auditory cortex, the part of the brain that processes sound, had been removed. The animals were then exposed to a sound at the same time that they received an electric shock. Even though the rats' brains could not register the sound, they all grew to fear it. The combination of the sound and shock had registered in the amygdala and created a lasting emotional response. This meant some kinds of information went straight to the amygdala and provoked an emotional response without the "thinking" involvement of the rest of the brain.

LeDoux's work shows that the thalamus sends some kinds of information directly to the amygdala for a fast, emotional response, instead of the relatively slow, cognitive response that the neocortex provides.

LeDoux posits that the rapid amygdala response is a survival mechanism, one that is found in every animal that has an amygdala. You are hiking in the mountains and the grizzly charges. The first response is to freeze momentarily; your brain is trying to work out exactly what is happening and how it should respond. The amygdala screams "RUN!" and your feet are moving before you realize it. This all occurs in milliseconds as the brain processes information from the senses.

This same mechanism is what prevents a shy child from introducing herself to a new student or raising her hand to answer a question in class. Researchers such as Kagan and LeDoux agree that much shy behavior is the result of an excitable amygdala. The shy child perceives danger in situations that an outgoing child does not. Her neocortex might realize logically that a new playmate is not a threat, but her amygdala—mediated by her self-talk—overrides it and takes over the forces of the adrenal system so that her face flushes, her palms sweat, and she desperately seeks a way out of this anxiety-provoking situation.

This discovery has tremendous applications for treating shy children. Even though we are talking about a biological process, there is overwhelming evidence that this process can be modified by consistent training. It helps us realize that temperamentally shy children need special types of instruction to recognize their feelings, to sense how their bodies react to those feelings, and to know how they can take control of the situation. Children who develop shyness later in life are held hostage by the same excitable amygdala, although it is believed that theirs has *learned* to overrespond to certain situations, thanks to the way memories are stored.

Memory is not stored in one particular place in the brain. Scientists are still researching the process of accumulating and retrieving memories, but it appears that there are several influences on how and where a memory is stored. The emotional state of a person when a memory is formed is one of those influences. Events that evoke a strong reaction from the amygdala appear to be stored in the amygdala itself, making the very strong sensory awareness that accompanies a fear reaction available instantly. Veterans clearly remember being pinned down by enemy fire fifty years after the event, but can't remember what they ate for dinner last week. This makes sense. To survive, we want those memories of incidents which were potentially dangerous to be the ones we can recall and react to the fastest. A child's reaction to a stressful situation will be colored by his memories of similar events, and memory is a powerful opponent to wrestle with.

Developmental Stages in the Brain

As a child grows and her brain develops, she uses the neocortex of her brain more. An infant responds to a stimulus: She cries from hunger or fear, she turns her head to nurse if something touches her cheek. A toddler knows how to get attention by throwing cereal on the floor and can sympathize with the feelings of others. The teenage brain, while nearly mature, is simultaneously developing new neural connections from education and experience while coping with the additional burden of hormones. Your child's ability to use the thinking part of her brain grows stronger as she matures, and so more can be done to help her override immediate shy responses.

The chapters in Part II on each developmental stage will give you specific information on how your child's age influences her shy behavior and how she an manage it.

THE USES OF UNDERSTANDING

Once you, as a parent, understand the variables that formed your shy child's personality, you can put the knowledge to work, first, by appreciating and honoring your child's uniqueness—coming as it does from a unique set of genetic combinations and life experiences—and, second, by separating her genetic birthright and experience from your own. Chances are that you identify yourself as either predominantly shy or predominantly nonshy. Though having either personality type in a parent can be an asset to a shy child, there are pitfalls that you should consider.

A Message to Nonshy Parents

So, you're baffled and exasperated. It is easy to guess what you're thinking. Why can't he just try harder? Why is he afraid of everything? Is he always going to be like this? Why is he so unhappy? Did we do something wrong? Maybe we should push him more. Maybe we should be stricter. Maybe we should force him to gut it out.

People who are not shy often cannot imagine what it's like. Much of the real pain, and occasionally terror, that is associated with feelings of shyness is internal. Remember the message from Chapter 2: The shy child is bombarded by negative self-talk, messages that increase his awareness of his surroundings and his doubts about what he is supposed to do. If you recorded a long tape of messages such as "Everyone is staring at you. They don't want you here. You look different. You're going to make a mistake. You don't know what you're doing. Everyone else is comfortable. You should have stayed home. You're incompetent," and then played that tape through the day so that only you could hear it as you tried to work and function socially, you would soon feel your confidence seep away. This is what it can feel like for your shy child in stressful situations.

As the biological and psychological underpinnings of shy-

ness become clearer, we are developing a better
works and doesn't work with shy children.

- *Pushing won't help.* Forcing your child to do what is terrifying him will only make the problem worse. There is a
  big difference between preparing your child for social situations with role-playing and forcing him out on the playground with no tools. You may be able to force yourself
  through stressful situations, but you must recognize that
  your child is different from you.

- *Your child is not acting this way to annoy you.* You might
  feel manipulated by your shy child, particularly if he
  promises one type of behavior and then does not follow
  through on it. It can be embarrassing to have all the other
  parents stare at you when your kid is the one who flees in
  tears, is struck speechless, or buries his head in your side
  and refuses to look at anyone. Your impatience and frustration are understandable, but remember that nobody
  would choose these feelings of self-doubt and anxiety.

- *Shyness does not mean your child's life is ruined.* Do not despair! Shyness is not a fatal illness, and it doesn't have to
  be a disability. Shyness is a complicated series of emotional
  reactions that can be moderated with practice so that your
  shy child becomes comfortable and confident. However,
  many aspects of a shy personality, such as sensitivity,
  strong observational skills, and the ability to work independently, are all enviable characteristics that will serve
  your child well if they are validated and respected.

- *You and your child can learn from each other.* Our children
  teach us from the day they are born. It is one of the many

unexpected and delightful surprises of parenting. There is much you can learn from your shy child, but you must be sensitive enough to find the best way to communicate with him. He sees the world through different eyes than you do. Given tolerance and understanding, you can *both* enjoy seeing it from each other's perspective.

A Message to Shy Parents

So, you think you know exactly how your child feels. You probably do have a handle on her feelings, but you must be careful not to *plant* fears or inhibit growth. If you were a shy child, you may be the best person in the world to parent a shy child. You understand her anxiety, and you know how important it is for her to feel secure so that she can develop an interior sense of balance and strength. On the other hand, shy parents can project their own fears and insecurities onto their child, making it difficult for the child to grow. Following are some stumbling blocks shy parents have encountered in parenting their shy children, with some general advice on how you can avoid them.

- *Babying won't help.* You will not help your child by protecting her from the world. In fact, sheltering her from social situations or those activities which trigger her anxieties will make her childhood difficult and could turn her into a miserable adult. However, your sensitivity can help you measure the rate at which your child moves. Shyness can be moderated by gentle, consistent exposure to other people. Your child must learn to increase her tolerance of others, much in the way she would develop calluses if she worked in the garden every day. She cannot build up the calluses if you never hand her the tools.

- *Recognize that your child is not you.* Having children allows us to relive our childhoods, for better or for worse. Do you remember feeling shy? It may be helpful for you to experience your memories. Jot down a few embarrassing moments from your youth. Note those times when you felt excruciatingly self-conscious, when you were sure the entire world was staring (maybe laughing) at you. Reconnecting with those emotions can help you understand how your child feels. It will also allow you to separate your personal distress from your child's. Remember that she may have gotten your shy gene, but it may be intensified or made less intense by her father's genetic makeup. And her experiences are inevitably different. If you seek to become more outgoing and self-confident, then you can do so alongside your child, but do not make the mistake of confusing her journey with your own.

- *Your child might be more comfortable than you are.* You are raising your child differently than your parents raised you; you are taking an active role in helping your child move beyond shyness so that she can live with comfort and confidence. You may be surprised at your own feelings of wistfulness when your hard work begins to pay off. When you teach your shy child to welcome the world, you will lose a small part of her, the dependent, insecure child who would turn to you for help. Let her surpass you. You have done it right when her social skills are better than yours.

- *You and your child can learn from each other.* Your own shyness can be a great asset for your shy child. You know, in a way a nonshy parent cannot, what it feels like to be shy. In turn, your shy child can show you a new way of approaching the world. She can guide you through her childhood, finding triumph instead of terror, success instead of shame. You will both win.

Finding Balance

While your goal is to make your shy child more comfortable with himself, to have him take control of his self-talk and to distinguish between a safe social situation and one that provokes an inappropriate emotional response, you do not want to squash all of the characteristics of shyness. Rather, you want your child to be able to discover who he really is under the layer of anxiety that has held him back. When reclaiming an overgrown garden, you don't rip out every single plant and start from bare earth. You clear the weeds and vines and look for the natural plantings that you can enhance.

Your shy child has several advantages over his outgoing peers. The expression "Still waters run deep" is a perfect description of the shy child's soul. Shy children are tremendous observers of the world around them; they may overreact to social signals, but they are way ahead of children who don't pick up on social signals at all. When they learn to interpret the signs of play and friendship, they become shrewd observers of human behavior. Their peers learn to pay attention when the shy child speaks because they know that, though he doesn't say much, what he contributes is important. These observational skills, and the ability to remain calm instead of bouncing off the walls in school, allow the shy child to learn a great deal.

Shy people often make the best friends. A shy child does

not develop friendships at the drop of a hat. When he allows himself to open up to a playmate, it is after a great deal of thought, and it requires untold sacrifice and discomfort. When a shy child makes a friend, it tends to be a long-standing, rewarding relationship. Shy children are loyal and tenacious; they keenly understand the value of friendships and go to great lengths to maintain them.

With the help of loving, engaged parents, shy children can grow up into tremendously accomplished adults. They weather the storms of personal self-doubt at an early age, and are more prepared for the buffeting winds of growth and development.

The Shy Label

We all identify traits in our children that help us to describe them to ourselves and others: She's the athletic one; he's the musical one. Labeling begins at birth as we scan our infant's face for clues about the soul within. Families trot out baby stories that "prove" the personality of a child, or point out those characteristics of a child that affirm his given role. Whom does he take after? What will he become? These attempts to pinpoint personality traits are inevitable to some degree and are a very human thing to do.

Shyness is a common label for parents to bestow on young children because they react shyly to new situations. Shyness is cute in a young child; adults find a blush, a bashful turn of the head, or a tentative smile appealing. Shyness may be adorable at four, but it is distracting at fourteen, and can be disabling at thirty-four.

The shy label, if it is pasted on in childhood and reinforced by parental expectations, is restrictive and unfair. Shyness waxes and wanes over time. The child who was shy through elementary school may have a great fifth-grade year and enter middle school feeling confident and self-assured. This growth can't happen if he continually hears that he is "the shy one."

Consider the experience of the nanny who accompanied a family on a beach vacation. As she sat with the family's seven-year-old son one day, she suggested that the boy approach the little boy playing alone on the blanket next to them.

"I can't," answered the boy. "I'm shy."

The nanny explained that was not a problem, everyone feels shy sometimes. "Just go over and introduce yourself," she suggested. "You could collect shells together."

The boy shook his head solemnly. "Mommy says that I'm shy and that's why I can't play with other kids. I'm too shy."

The problem with labeling a child as shy does not mean you should never suggest to your child that she is shy. If you have determined that shyness is a stumbling block for her in social and school situations, then it is necessary to talk openly with her about it. The trick is to do it consciously and with a positive approach. Focus on the good qualities in your child and make a big deal of them. Your image of your child is folded into her image of herself. If you exhibit your anxiety about her shyness, she will mirror your fears. If you talk frankly about it and help her accept that her shyness is part of a total, wonderful package, she will be less stressed about it too, and more open to the possibility that she can use her shyness to her own best advantage.

The Family's Role

Another complication with labeling children as shy can be that other family members pick up on the label and reinforce a negative self-image related to it. There is nothing wrong with grandparents, aunts, cousins, uncles, and other nonshy children in the family accepting and honoring your shy child's personality the same way you do. But they must be brought along in the understanding that shyness is a style, not a disorder, and that people can change and adapt as they pass developmental stages.

Siblings Shy children often develop strong bonds with their siblings. The emotional energy that a nonshy child would expend on friends is poured out to siblings by a shy child. Having a brother or sister who understands the shy child provides comfort, acceptance, and a stronger sense of self-worth.

An outgoing sibling can be an invaluable teacher, even if the outgoing child is younger than the shy child. As a parent, you can initiate conversations during which the shy and nonshy siblings compare notes about a social situation, like a family party, school concert, or trip to the crowded mall. An uninhibited sibling offers a different view of the world: "Those people weren't staring at you; they were looking at the store window behind you," "Everyone hates to talk to teachers after class, but it can help you get a better grade, so do it!" or "You don't have to get permission; just tell them that you want to play." Siblings are loving tutors.

Grandparents, Aunts, and Uncles The extended family can make a tremendous contribution to the life of a shy child. They have the perspective that often allows them to value each child as an individual. They are less concerned with a child's ability to fit in. Grandparents, especially, having experienced the growth of their own children, are more confident in the knowledge that children find their own place in the fullness of time.

Grandparents can afford to be patient. Their lives are not necessarily as affected by the hurried pace of modern life. A shy child visiting a grandparent's house is allowed the time and space she needs. The unchanging environment of the grandparent's home, the calm pace of life, unconditional love, and understanding—they add up to a warm, accepting sanctuary for the shy child.

Gretchen was able to spend two weeks at her grandparents' house in the Adirondack Mountains when she was eight years old. Her days were spent helping her grandmother cook or work on her pottery or watching her grandfather in his wood shop. Each afternoon she and her grandfather would walk to the corner store for bread or ice cream. The walks were long and silent. Her grandfather sometimes pointed to a bird or flower, but usually they walked hand in hand, enjoying the serenity of the woods around them.

For the rest of her childhood and now as an adult, Gretchen used that memory as a spiritual retreat when she felt anxious. When she felt overwhelmed by the world, she could retreat for a few minutes into the memory and come back refreshed.

Grandparents who do not live close by can play an important role with letters or e-mail. Talking on the telephone is hard for some shy children. Getting a letter is ideal. First, it is private. Reading a letter is an experience that the child can control. Once the child has learned to write, he may find it easier to express his feelings on paper. Regular correspondence from grandparents can be like having a cheerleader in the shy child's corner.

Parents should enlist the aid of grandparents and other members of the extended family when they decide to help their shy child learn to be more comfortable dealing with the world. The first step is for a frank discussion of how the family sees the child, and how the child's shyness interferes with his happiness and development. Parents can then explain what the family can do to help the child cope. Using the checklists in Chapters 5 through 10 may be helpful. Do not be afraid to insist on basic guidelines: helping the child identify his feelings, not labeling him "shy," being supportive not smothering, loving not protective.

CHAPTER SUMMARY

This chapter explored where shyness comes from: inherited shy tendencies, and the inhibited behaviors that develop in response to trauma, as well as what goes on in the body and brain of a shy child when he is feeling anxious and unsure. Here are the key points to remember:

1. Twenty percent of children are born with shy tendencies.

2. Another two out of five children will, at some point in their lives, exhibit shy behaviors in response to something going on in their world.

3. Understanding how traumas can affect your child is a step toward helping him cope with his anxiety.

4. Knowing how the brain reacts can assist in understanding the biological basis for anxiety.

5. Nonshy parents must respect their child's personality and not try to bully him into something he is not.

6. Shy parents cannot always assume they understand what their child is experiencing.

7. Families must honor each child for who she is, and avoid labeling. Every member in the extended family can be a valuable ally of the shy child.

8. Whether a child is temperamentally shy, or shy because of life events, he deserves balance in his soul: the chance to enjoy his strengths in observation, perception, and thoughtfulness with a growing self-confidence.

Chapter 4

HOW CAN I HELP MY CHILD?

By now it is clear that shyness is a personality style with many positive aspects, but one that can hinder a child's development and happiness if it prevents him from having a normal social life. We have seen that one child out of five is born with shy tendencies, and that others develop shyness in response to life experiences. Feelings of anxiety have a biological basis, but they can be modified and controlled by changing behavior and regulating self-talk.

This chapter presents the blueprint for working with your shy child. You will learn how to strengthen and enrich your relationship with her, how to establish effective communication, and what kinds of activities will desensitize her to anxiety-provoking situations. In Part II, you will find that you can apply the principles described in the following pages to the challenges presented by specific age groups.

LISTENING WITH LOVE

Most parents are great talkers. We can get our kids out the door in the morning, remind them to wear their jackets, make sure homework is finished and teeth are brushed. We can tell them how we think they should behave and lecture them when they have let us down. We lead busy, highly structured lives that require energy, organization, and a parent in charge to direct the action. Our children have calluses on their ears from all the talking we direct at them, and our own listening skills have withered from lack of use.

Before we do any type of shyness work with our children, we must enhance our relationship with them. Listening implies love.

Your First Task

Your first activity is to have a conversation with your shy child. That sounds easy, doesn't it? But there are some ground rules. First, it cannot be an interrogation. Asking what your child did in school doesn't count. Neither does criticizing what his room looks like or reminding him to practice the trombone. Second, the conversation must center on a mutual interest, something you and your child have in common or both enjoy doing. It may be a sports team you both like, the family plans for the weekend, a television program or movie, a hobby you enjoy.

Schedule some time alone with your child: one parent, one child, without distractions or interruptions. Perhaps you can take a walk together or work in the yard. The conversation only needs to last for fifteen minutes. The first time you try this, fifteen minutes may seem like a very long time, but it will get easier with practice. Don't worry if you feel awkward, or if your first attempts seem fumbling and silly. You have years of practice telling your child what to do. It may take a little while to get used to listening to him. The goal is to have at least one fifteen-minute relaxed conversation about a mutual interest every day. You may be surprised at what a delightful improvement this small change will make in your relationship with your child.

From Talk to Trust

Your shy child may have already made a habit of subduing her feelings before they ever reach a level where she can even acknowledge them. You need to lay a firm foundation of trust to get to the place where your child is ready to share her feelings with you and work to tackle what makes her anxious.

Of course, you already have a relationship with your child. You love your child and are concerned about her welfare and happiness. You are obviously involved enough to realize that her shyness is interfering with her growth, and you have gone to the trouble to discover what you can do to help. But just as your child has developed habits in regard to her feelings, chances are you have too. You may have gotten used to her silence and acquiescence when you tell her what *you* think she should do or what *you* thought of the movie. If you have other children who are more vocal about their feelings and are more demanding of your attention, your shy child's quietness has probably seemed a blessing, one that is easy to take for granted. Even if your shy child is the most cuddly and physically demonstrative of your children, establishing a genuine relationship of trust in regard to expressing feelings and opinions may be a surprisingly complex task.

We could all stand to improve our relationships with our children. The structure of our society chips away at the natural bonds between parent and child. Many parents must hand their child to caregivers when the child is six weeks old. From that point on, contact is hampered by time constraints and the need to get things done. We feed our children, clothe them, work hard to provide for them. As they grow older, we meet with teachers and drive our children to soccer practice, Scouts, ballet, and the mall. We make sure teeth are brushed and beds are made. But we don't hang out much with our kids. Once they grow beyond the block-stacking years, we don't get down on the floor and play with them. It is our loss as much as theirs.

All children need easy, comfortable access to their parents. The difference between outgoing children who are in touch with and vocal about their feelings is that they know how to demand such access, and they know instinctively how to meet their parents halfway in terms of conversation and social interaction with them. Shy children, to one degree or another, wait for signals from their parents. If those signals don't come, they either keep waiting, give up in frustration, or take out their (unnamed and unacknowledged) frustration in sudden temper tantrums or other destructive behavior. It is also logical that some shy children, unlike their outgoing counterparts, do not know how to keep a conversation going, even with their parents.

The Second Task

What kinds of activities can you enjoy with your child? Watching your child play basketball and cheering wildly on the sidelines is good, but it is not good enough for developing the kind of relationship you need to help him with his shyness. *Playing* basketball with your child is what's needed. You want to come up with interactive activities that you will both enjoy. Some families keep a card table standing to hold an airplane model or puzzle-in-progress. (Don't have the television on while you are working on these projects!) Another family builds birdhouses together. Can you start a crafts project for holiday gift-giving? Are there board games your child loves to play, but for which you never seem to have the time? One mother has a lifelong game of Crazy Eights going with her daughter. They keep score in a book that is already ten years old. For regular opportunities to talk, nothing beats planting a garden with your child—let her decide what goes in it—and setting aside time to weed and talk each week.

Play with your child. Make play as important, more important, than work. Make time for it, anticipate it with joy, dress properly for it. When it's playtime, put on your jeans or sweatpants and get on the floor with him. Make noises, be a car, be a dinosaur. Your child will be delighted and you will get back more love and positive behavior than you ever dreamed possible.

Dolls are wonderful tools for interaction. It doesn't matter if your child plays with baby dolls, Barbie dolls, stuffed animals, puppets, or action figures; if you can get involved in that play, you will learn an enormous amount about the inner workings of your child's mind. When they play with dolls, children act out the conflicts of their own world, and express feelings they may be uncomfortable voicing in direct conversation. Young children are not as verbal as adults. You can learn more from direct observation of behavior than by questioning.

What does playing with your child have to do with shyness? Everything. The family unit is usually the safest, most functional place for a shy child, so it is the best place to work on shyness issues. But too often, the parent-child relationship dribbles away into one of giving and receiving orders. To help him come out of his shell, you must prepare the ground, solidify your bonds with your child, before you can expect him to open up about his thoughts and feelings.

The Power of the Rocking Chair. If your child's shyness is significantly interfering with her development, you need to make time to hold and rock her. Invite your younger child into your lap for a cuddle. An older child can be cajoled or teased in a friendly way: "You're not too old to sit on Mom's lap, are you?" Ten minutes a day of rocking will help you connect with your child and help strengthen her. Even if the child is as big as you are, she will respond to the familiar, loving sensation of a parent's arms holding her close. If you have a teenager who would rather chew glass than sit in your lap, arrange to spend time together sitting on the couch; drag out family pictures to share, or show her something in a magazine that will interest her.

Ten-year-old Ashley's parents were stunned at the difference they saw in their intensely shy daughter when they concentrated on building a relationship with her. She was not a problem child. She was not in any trouble. Teachers didn't really notice her much, and her grades were good enough. She preferred to spend time alone in her room, but she had never acted out. She was just quiet. When her parents intentionally spent time with her, cuddled with her, and developed common interests that parents and daughter could enjoy and discuss, they reported that "it was like turning on a lamp." Their daughter had more to say to them than they had ever imagined she carried within! As the relationship strengthened, she blossomed. Once she could share her thoughts and feelings with her parents, she found she could share them with friends and teachers as well. The foundation that her parents constructed allowed her to become more secure, and then face the rest of the world with an eagerness for new experiences.

THE MAGIC OF ART

Children constantly offer us clues to what they are thinking and feeling; we must be clever enough to notice the hints and interpret them correctly. Artwork is a trail of bread crumbs that will lead you to discovering how your child sees herself.

Pay attention to your child's drawings. Where does she stand in relation to the others when she draws herself? If she constantly draws herself as an isolated figure, far away from a group of other relatives, or friends, or classmates, then there is something to be concerned about. She may draw herself in an aggressive posture toward someone, or she may draw a person who constantly teases her as much larger than she.

When you talk to your child about her art, you must be calm and interested, but not overly concerned. If you grew up in the 1970s, you may remember a television detective named Columbo. This seemingly befuddled, rumpled character always solved the case by asking obvious questions and playing a little dumb. That's a good posture for you to strike when you talk to your child about her artwork. Ask her to tell you what is happening in the picture. Say "I don't understand, tell me again." Keep your face and body language neutral. If you act worried or upset about what your child is drawing or telling you, she will shut down and you will lose a valuable communication outlet. Do not ask her to tell you what she's feeling. That doesn't work.

You will start to see patterns in her art, patterns that will be reflected in other types of play, like dolls or pretend games with siblings. Is she always being yelled at? Does she always return to the same themes, or use negative self-talk to scold or criticize? These are patterns of self-evaluation and thinking. This is how your child sees the world, and where she sees herself in it. Be careful not to take one drawing or an overheard conversation with a teddy bear out of context and become unduly alarmed. You are looking for the forest here, not the trees.

Be aware that your child is observing you just as you are observing her. If you look bored, insincere, or you overreact when she says something that disturbs you, she will change her behavior based on your reaction. You want to maintain a neutral, interested stance when you talk with your child, or observe her play.

Once you have grown comfortable talking to your child about her art, it is time for *you* to pick up the crayon. You are going to sit at the table next to her and draw. Don't worry; no art teacher will be grading you. It doesn't matter if your dogs look like cows or if your houses are architectural nightmares. Drawing with your child validates the experience; it shows her you think art is fun, important, and a good way to spend time. It is a peaceful activity. Once she is used to your presence (and your dog-cows) she will open up more, talking about her pictures as she is creating them.

One first-grade girl who loved to swing at recess continually drew the swing set on the playground. However, she was never on the swing. Even though the school rule was that children could only swing for five minutes, she couldn't bring herself to tell other kids their time was up. (Her teachers took the attitude that if she wouldn't ask for her turn on the swings, then she must not want to swing.)

Her mother decided to work on the swing set problem. Sitting next to her daughter, she drew a picture of one child swinging and a little girl waiting her turn. Talking aloud as she drew, she sketched out different scenarios. In one, the waiting girl said, "It's my turn. You have to get off now," and the kid on the swings jumped off. In another, the kid on the swings ignored the little girl, and she had to yell loudly, "It's my turn to swing!" The woman's daughter started to help her mother. They both drew the swing set scene over and over, talking about different positive and negative options, what the two children might say to each other, how the little girl could react. The mother and daughter repeated this over the course of several weeks, until the daughter came home one morning with a wide grin. She told the other child to get off the swings when her time was up and the other child listened! For the first time since school started, the girl was able to swing at recess.

DRAWING OUT THE PROBLEM

1. Identify a shy scenario that is causing problems, one that you see in your child's artwork or see her reenacting in play.

2. Divide several sheets of paper into blocks, as if you were drawing a comic strip.

3. Draw the scenario, talking out loud to describe what you are drawing.

4. Draw optional solutions to the problems—good ones and bad ones. Ask your child for input, "What could happen next?" Give your child the chance to contribute to your picture and be prepared to surrender the paper to her if she wants to take it over.

5. Always end your art time on a positive note, with your child drawn smiling and in control.

6. Repeat this session many times over weeks or months. Repetition is crucial to break old habits and dissolve a negative self-talk. New options will crop up. As your child tries the new behavior, it may have unforeseen consequences she needs to learn how to handle.

7. Keep the pictures—file them away or post the best examples on the refrigerator.

THE DAILY DISCUSSION

Give yourself several weeks to enrich the relationship with your child. Keeping a diary may be helpful. We schedule everything else in our lives; there is nothing wrong with blocking out "alone time" with your child on your calendar. There may be some false starts and bad days, but once you and your child have gotten into a healthy pattern of openness and time doing things together, you can start working on his shyness issues.

These are the five components to shyness work:

- Observation;

- Daily discussion;

- Scripting;

- Role-playing; and

- Reviewing.

You have already started observing. You will, of course, continue doing this: making time to draw together, to talk about your child's art, to play and pretend. Beyond that, you will start an intentional daily discussion.

For some parents, the daily discussion will be completely natural, an outgrowth of their existing communication style. For others, it will be more of an effort. The point of the daily discussion is to discover what is going on in your child's life. You accomplish this with open-ended questions, questions that cannot be answered with a yes or no. You could start by asking your child's opinion about something. The conversation should proceed in a nonthreatening fashion. Your goal is to work your way to the point where your child will openly discuss his shyness issues with you.

You can also use the daily discussion to review the day with your child. You may need to be more tuned in to the activities within her classroom than you currently are. If neces-

sary, meet with your child's teacher to get an outline of topics, assignments, projects, and assemblies. Journalists know
that the best question to ask is one to which they already have
the answer. You are a reporter who must seek out more than
the concrete details of the day; you want to explore the emotions and motivation under the surface.

As your child opens up about his feelings and the awkward
situations he dreads, treat it in a matter-of-fact fashion. Don't
overreact. You must be careful about your word choice,
avoiding judgmental or dismissive language. Shy children are
auditorily as well as visually hypervigilant. They clue in to
every nuance in your voice.

Be thoughtful about the timing of the discussion. You
know best which time periods are stress-filled and when the
family is more relaxed. Our culture is plagued by a lack of time
for our children. If you have to make changes in your life to
carve out fifteen minutes to talk to your child every day, then
do it right now. It is the wisest investment you will ever make.

The idea of having time with you every day will appeal to
most children, whether they are young or old. Older children,
though, especially teenagers, often require more detailed information surrounding the nature of the daily discussion. That is,
the purpose behind it might need to be more blatantly expressed
than with younger children. For guidelines, see Chapter 7.

Children of any age might balk sometimes at having regularly scheduled meetings. For the most part, if you make it
clear that you are committed to having time alone every day,
it will soon become as routine as eating breakfast. If your child
questions the process at first, simply let her know this is something you want to do. If she has some days when she feels too
rotten or is too tired to engage with you, then be sensitive to
that. Just don't let too many days in a row pass like that.

The "Daily Discussion" sections in Chapters 7 through 9 will help you devise activities and topics for daily discussion with your child which are keyed to his particular age and level of development.

THE PRECOCIOUS CHILD

Some children, particularly only children, can come across as highly verbal and pseudomature. They spent a great deal of time watching and listening to adults and they are great mimics. Don't let it fool you. Emotionally, even the most precocious eight-year-old is still eight years old. Don't let a highly verbal child control discussions about his shyness and feed you the answers he thinks you want. To really know what is going on in his heart, observe his play, participate in his pretend world, and study his artwork. That is where you will find the truth about his feelings.

EXPLORING THE SHY SCENARIO

As you regularly listen to your child, play with him, and observe his art and play patterns, you will understand what his shy scenarios are. The shy scenario is any situation that makes your child feel and act shy. Your child cannot "fix" all his scenarios with a single blow. The two of you will tackle his scenarios one at a time, starting with a relatively simple situation that you feel he can master, such as greeting a child you know is friendly, or checking out his own library books.

Most shy scenarios can be scripted; they can be broken down into scene after scene much as a director might describe the action in a screenplay. In your discussion time with your child, ask him to script the scenario. Be careful not to interrogate—be playful! All you are looking for is a blow-by-blow description—first this happened, and then that happened. Keep your face and voice neutral as he talks. If you react in a judgmental way by frowning, offering sympathy, or criticizing, he will not be able to trust you and nothing will be accomplished.

You may be able to see how your child could have behaved differently. Resist the temptation to tell him what he did wrong. Rather, ask him in what other ways he could have thought or reacted. You want to keep the focus narrow. Target one aspect of his behavior he could have changed. The goal in working with your shy child is to offer him simple, manageable tasks that are so small he can't help but succeed. Each success is the foundation stone for the next.

Here is an example of how a parent can learn the details of a shy scenario:

Child: "I had some trouble at lunch today, again."
Parent: "Tell me what happened at lunch."
Child: "Jason took my cookie again."
Parent: "Tell me how it happened."
Child: "I was sitting at my seat and Jason was across from me."
Parent: "Who was near you?"
Child: "I sit on the end, so there's nobody on that side. Kyra sits on the other side and Jenna sits next to her. Robert sits next to Jason. They're friends."
Parent: "What did Jason say to you?"
Child: "I don't know. He just talks to Robert and then he looks at me and takes my cookie. I don't

know what to do. It's not fair. It was a peanut butter cookie today."

Parent: "Where were the lunch monitors when this happened?"

Child: "I don't know. Somewhere."

Parent: "When did this happen?"

Child: "After Jason finished his potato chips. He was still hungry."

Parent: "Peanut butter and potato chips. Yuk! What did you do when he took your cookie?"

Child: "Nothing."

Parent: "You did a really good job describing what happened to me. Now I can see what you are up against. Let's brainstorm and come up with a few things you can try the next time this happens."

Scripting

Once you understand what is happening, you must identify small changes your child can make in his reaction. Maintain a relaxed, playful attitude with your child as the two of you come up with alternative outcomes. He is already stressed, both from the incident, and from reliving the feelings as he recounts it. It's up to you to break the tension. You can call it "The What-If Game," or "Imagine That . . .".

Parent: "What if your cookie came to life when Jason grabbed it, and it bit his thumb and he ran around the cafeteria hollering and was sent to the principal's office?"

Child: (giggling)

Parent: "What if a superhero flew into the cafeteria and yelled at Jason for being a cookie snatcher and gave you a medal for "Bravery in the Face of a Horrible Cookie Snatcher?"

Child: (more giggling)

Parent: "What if you looked at Jason's eyes when he took your cookie and told him no?"

Child: "I could never do that!"

Parent: "What could you do?"

Child: "I could hide my cookie on my lap."

Parent: "That would make it harder for him to grab it. Do you think you could look at him too? He doesn't have laser eyes that fry your brain, does he? Could you give him a 'Don't You Even Think About My Cookie' stare while you enjoy your cookie? What would that stare look like?"

Child: (glares and giggles)

Role-playing and Rehearsing New Scenarios

Once you and your child have scripted alternatives to the shy scenario, it is important that you act them out with him. This might feel awkward for you both; again, a sense of humor and atmosphere of playfulness will go a long way toward making you feel comfortable and helping the lesson sink in. Your child will slip in the world of pretend more easily if he senses that you are having fun. Nobody is going to judge your performance. If you feel odd, just imagine what your child feels when trapped in the scenario itself.

There are many variations to rehearsing alternative scenarios. If you have your child take on the role of someone other than himself, you will hear him act out what he thinks others are thinking about him. Switch roles with your child from time to time. You can use props to help get into the feel. Visiting the site where the scenario takes place and performing your role-playing there would be extremely helpful.

As you get into role-playing, you may realize that the alternative scenario doesn't work. Perhaps you are pushing too hard. Reexamine—how can you break down the changes into smaller steps? A child who feels intimidated while walking between classes might be overwhelmed at your suggestion that she smile at students she doesn't know. You could start by having her select eye-level visual reference points so that she walks along with her head up instead of staring at the floor. Remember—small steps are successful steps. Never fear stopping a session and returning to it later following careful thought and planning.

Different Ages, Different Games. With children younger than five, you may want to present role-playing as "pretending." In your child's pretend world, anything can happen. Your child can have a different name or become an elephant or sprout wings that come in handy when he wants to get out of a tight spot. Again, the key is to give him a chance to work through a situation that makes him anxious, and to give him alternative resolutions, broken down into small, manageable steps.

Teenagers may roll their eyes and sigh at the first suggestion of role-playing, but don't let that stop you. They are actually quite good at this. Your playful, relaxed attitude will give them permission to get into the game. Use different voices, pretend to be a Shakespearean actor, exaggerate your role, and let yourself have fun. If your teenager is extremely resistant, then offer a compromise. Let him try to work through a particular shy scenario his way. If he is not seeing any improvement in his comfort level after an agreed-to period of time, then he promises to try it your way.

Adolescents and school-age children can also use visualizations as a form of role-playing. This should not take the place of actually acting out alternative scenarios, but it makes a great companion to them. Your child should practice visualizations when he is calm and relaxed; just before falling asleep is a perfect time for them. He should relax his body and take slow, regular breaths. Once he is settled, have him visualize the shy scenario with a positive outcome that you have scripted with him ahead of time. Have him pay attention to the tension of his body. He may find his hands balling into fists, or his stomach clenching as he plays out the scene in his mind. Remind him to breathe deeply and regularly, easing his way through the scenario and always ending on a positive note. Visualization is a powerful tool that is used by many professional athletes to improve their game and help them maintain a winning attitude. It belongs in the tool chest of your shy child as well.

MY CHILD'S SELF-TALK MESSAGES
AND SHY SCENARIOS

After a few weeks of observing and playing with your child, you should start to get a sense of his self-talk messages and the type of situations that provokes negative self-talk. Write down what he is telling himself and why. Note his shy scenarios and the alternatives that he creates.

Using Failure—Revising and Rewriting Scenarios

Part of helping your child take control of her shy scenarios is acknowledging that things may not go as planned. Once you have scripted a reasonable alternative, ask her to imagine what can go wrong. Do not make fun of her if she presents unrealistic disasters; instead, say, "I never thought about that happening. What else?" Your child may become anxious while talking about her scenario, particularly when she thinks about all the things that can go wrong. Shy kids are great "catastrophizers." By experiencing the anxiety at home with you, she has the chance to control the emotions and begin to build up the callus that will ultimately protect her from anxiety.

Looking at possible failures presents you with a terrific teaching opportunity. As your child enumerates all the things that can go wrong, you can work with her to develop responses that she will use the rest of her life: how to deal with bullies, how to express anger, how to get a teacher's attention, how to introduce herself to strangers, how to shake hands, how to get out of a boring conversation politely—some kids may pick these skills up by observation, but your shy child needs you to explain them.

It is absurd to think that you must have all the answers at your fingertips all the time. You don't know everything—no one does—and you teach your child another lesson by being honest about your limitations. If your child presents you with a difficult situation that doesn't have an easy solution, be honest and admit "That's a tough one—let me think about it for a while." Talk to other parents, contact your child's guidance counselor, go to the library and read up on the topic. When you talk to your child, explain how you researched your solution so that she can learn from your experience.

You should plan on spending at least an hour a week working with your child on his shy scenarios: scripting, role-playing, and reviewing. This is in addition to your fifteen-minute daily discussion, and whatever time you spend playing with your child and observing him. Some problems may require an intense burst of time and effort; your child finds out he must give an oral presentation in a week, for example. If you are not under a time crunch, don't force daily sessions. Your child needs time to digest what the two of you are working on.

Giving Credit Where Credit Is Due

Remember to maintain a neutral tone of voice and facial expressions as you review and rewrite scenarios. This is particularly important as your child reports something that went poorly. You are deeply invested in helping your child succeed and it is easy to take his missteps personally. You do not want your disappointment to cause him to dress up the truth or lie about his experiences just to please you.

Equally important is encouraging your child to take credit when things go well. Shy children tend to discount success. Parents of shy children will often hear statements like, "They didn't really want me to play with them" or "He didn't mean that; he hates me." Shy children will never be accused of hogging the limelight; they are unassuming, not boastful. A crucial part of shyness work is teaching children to take credit for their victories, to help them see how their changed behavior leads others to treat them differently and themselves to positive self-talk, pride, and assurance.

Watch your own language. Self-effacement and extreme modesty may be part of your family culture. Do you have a hard time taking credit for your achievements? Do you blush or downplay what you've done when someone compliments you? Are you quick to bring up the participation of others and reduce or ridicule your own role? Think of the impact this has on your shy child. By not taking credit for your own accomplishments, you model destructive behavior and send the message that it is bad to feel good about yourself and your work. You don't intend it that way, but that is how the shy child sees it. There is a world of difference between a loud-mouthed, cocky braggart and a person who is confident and appropriately proud of herself. Make sure you can provide a healthy model of self-assurance for your child.

Setting Goals

You need to set two types of goals: long- and short-term. Keep the long-term goals to yourself; there is no need to burden a shy child with your vision of her future social skills. You may have chosen inappropriate, unrealistic, or even insufficient goals, and if you share them with your child, it will be extremely hard to revise them. If you want, keep track of your goals in a diary or journal. Revisit them occasionally as your child progresses and make any necessary adjustments. The ultimate goal is to help your child become comfortable with herself and confident in social situations.

One area where long-term goals is crucial is schoolwork. Some shy children are expert at procrastinating because the thought of some kinds of homework, like working on a group project, interviewing strangers, making phone calls, or speaking in front of a group, is so painful. They can even fool themselves into believing that they really don't have to do it. The result is always heartbreak—either a storm of emotion the night before the assignment is due, or a poor grade and a phone call from the teacher.

Be alert to the requirements of your child's class. Talk to the guidance counselor and teacher at the same time, explaining that your child is working on developmental issues that require you to be more aware of class assignments than might otherwise be the case. As soon as an assignment is given, sit down with your child and break it down into small tasks. Schedule these tasks on a family calendar and follow through to make sure they are being accomplished on time.

Short-term shyness goals must be broken up into tiny pieces in the same way. The goals will depend on the scenario and severity of your child's shyness. One fourteen-year-old who could not bring himself to talk to or even look at anyone outside his family set as his goal walking into a room with other people and keeping his breathing under control. He didn't have to start a conversation or look anyone in the eye— he just had to stand in the room, maintain awareness of how he felt, and focus on breathing normally. This was a manageable goal, one that gave him a feeling of success and had the added benefit of relaxing his body.

Shy children can give off unfriendly signals; for them, learning how to appear open can be broken down into tiny steps that add up to a great reward. Your child may want to set a short-term goal of walking into a room with a neutral expression instead of frowning or learn to keep his hands out of his pocket. Both girls and boys hide behind their hair; have them set a goal of finding a hairstyle they like that will show their face to the world. Adolescents can use bad hygiene as a pungent avoidance technique. With a child like this, you cannot set daily showers as a short-term goal. But you can start with clean hands and daily face washing. Then you move to clean clothes every day. The pace must be determined by your child. If it seems excruciatingly slow to you, take heart in the progress itself and don't fret about the pace.

A Small Step for Your Child, a Giant Leap for His Confidence. We don't want to put kids in situations for which they are not developmentally ready. Forcing them beyond what they are prepared for will cause significant levels of anxiety and distress. The biggest mistake parents make is to expect too much too soon. Some parents want their shy children to leap from point A to point F and skip all the steps in between. This is as understandable as it is regrettable, and is another sign that parents do not fully understand the nature of shyness. Every time a shy child evaluates a social situation negatively, the bonds between the event and the child's discomfort strengthen. The stronger the bonds become, the harder they are to break.

The desire to change must start with your child. If you are the only one who wants your child to be more outgoing, it will not work. The parents of an eleven-year-old boy brought in for counseling insisted that he wanted to work on his anxieties. The truth of the matter was that he had been tricked into getting in the car and had no idea his parents had arranged for him to meet with a therapist. He was angry and betrayed, and refused to speak to the therapist. His parents could no longer be trusted. After that day, the boy never wanted to get in the car; he couldn't believe his own mother and father. Parents sometimes make difficult decisions out of love on the premise that the ends justify the means.

Machiavelli does not apply to children. The means must justify the end; every step of the path to self-confidence must be taken with compassion and trust. Keep the steps small and gentle.

Think of standing barefoot next to a small child; visualize how big your feet are compared to hers. When the child walks, she takes steps that are just right for her. If she tries to walk in your footsteps, she struggles, jumps, or fails. Don't force your child to work through her shyness issues at your pace. Help her find her own pace. Every successful experience chisels away at the negative bonds. You will not err by making too small a step.

A WORD ABOUT "SHOULD"

One last comment about expectations: Make every effort to avoid using "should" when you are dealing with your child's shyness issues. Saying something like "You should be able to talk to the neighbor's boy" or "You should be able to ask for help" may seem innocuous, but sentences like this are destructive to your child and cloud your judgment. There is a difference between internally setting long-term goals of happiness and comfort for your child and short-term goals of small-step success, and harshly measuring her against an arbitrary social yardstick.

You are your child's safety net, the one person she can trust in a world that feels hostile and unwelcoming. She looks to you for comfort, assurance, and help. The way you react to her behavior and emotions can set her on a course for a life of worry and pain, or a fulfilled, enriched adulthood. You would never dream of feeding your child a diet of cod liver oil, unflavored oat bran, and protein powder. Make sure you nurture with an abundant diet of love, patience, and compassion.

These are the minimum daily requirements needed to help a shy child grow.

CHAPTER SUMMARY

1. Parents need to develop better listening skills.

2. Parents who spend interactive, fun time on activities with their children have stronger, more loving relationships.

3. There must be strong relationship bonds between parent and child before shyness work can begin.

4. Parents can observe a great deal about their child's self-talk, shyness issues, and sense of self-worth by observing the child's artwork.

5. Parents can use drawing and playing together as opportunities to work out problematic shy scenarios with their child.

6. Scheduling a fifteen-minute daily discussion between parent and child reinforces trust and understanding.

7. Once you understand your child's shy scenarios, you should spend at least an hour a week helping the child to think of alternative scenarios, practice role-playing, and anticipate problems.

8. Children can learn many important social skills by reviewing their shy scenarios with their parents.

9. Parents don't need to have all the answers; by sharing how they turn to others for help, they model important behavior for their children.

10. Shy children must learn how to take credit for their own successes. Parents should make sure that they know how to take credit for their own work and can show children how to do so appropriately.

11. Setting small, manageable short-term goals is crucial for working through shyness issues. Parents must keep long-term goals to themselves and be patient with their child's slow, steady progress.

Part Two

AGE-APPROPRIATE STRATEGIES FOR HELPING YOUR CHILD MANAGE SHYNESS

Chapter 5

BIRTH TO AGE TWO

It is never too early to begin teaching your shy child good socialization habits. Even infants who have shy characteristics can modify their natural tendencies if they are exposed to healthy social situations on a regular basis. The attitude and behavior of parents strongly affect how a shy infant or toddler responds to others. If parents react with anxiety whenever their shy child shows fear, then the child's impression that strange places, people, and things are dangerous will be reinforced, and he will become more inhibited. At the other extreme, parents who ignore a shy child's distress, or who don't recognize it when he feels overwhelmed, can make a child feel completely at the mercy of an unpredictable world. Again, the result is a child who withdraws.

This chapter will explain appropriate levels of socialization for shy infants and toddlers and will show parents how to help their children get off to a healthy relationship with the rest of the world.

EARLY SIGNS OF A SHY PERSONALITY STYLE

The idea that a baby is clay, waiting for the hands of his parents to mold him, is generally considered to be outdated. Your child came into the world with his personality intact, just as surely as he was born with ten fingers and ten toes. It is true, however, that the kinds of experiences he has and the way he is taught to react to those experiences can have an influence on how his inborn personality develops.

When personality causes complications in the social world, then some modification is desirable. If a child is naturally aggressive to the extent that he causes harm to himself or others, for example, his environment and upbringing can help him temper his aggressive behavior and lead him to use his natural tendencies in creative and productive ways. Likewise, a child who is so passive as to be easily taken advantage of needs nurturing to become more assertive. The trick in either case is to work within the framework of the inborn personality so as not to thwart a child's nature, which can cause a lifetime of stress.

It is fairly easy to spot a shy ten-year-old. But is it possible to recognize shy tendencies in babies? There are a few signs that indicate you are living with a child whose inclination, like 20 percent of babies, is toward a more inhibited, shy, introspective view of the world.

The Watcher

Shy babies sometimes remind adults of tiny owls. Their arms and legs are more still, and their eyes intently examine everything that goes on around them. They do not respond physically to what they see, but rather seem to be waiting until they have fully assessed the situation before they react. When presented with a new toy, for example, they are less likely to reach for it than outgoing babies. They may startle more easily and react more strongly to unfamiliar smells, sounds, and people.

Shy babies respond well to structure, daily routines that they anticipate and enjoy. They are more likely to become distressed when the routine is disrupted. When several new activities, many new faces, or a surfeit of new toys are presented at once, the shy baby may appear to withdraw or become agitated. While an outgoing child might seem energized and excited during an extended-family Christmas celebration, for example, a shy baby may become very quiet, may fall asleep, or may even fly into a temper.

The Time Bomb

Parents of shy babies are sometimes embarrassed by their children's public behavior. They compare their fussy, hard-to-please baby with others who seem constantly to be embracing new experiences with a smile. Parents sometimes feel their sensitive child is like dynamite waiting to explode. They try (in vain) to keep the house completely quiet while the "time bomb" naps. They run around trying to find the exact right combination of toys, food, and activity that their child requires. When they don't get it right, they suffer through hours of a crying baby and feel like failures.

Parents who have a baby who is easily overstimulated first deserve a pat on the back, and perhaps the offer of free baby-sitting so they can go out to dinner. While they enjoy a quiet, peaceful meal, they can brainstorm about the best way to treat the child, respecting the sensitive temperament, while helping the child adjust to the real world. They can examine their routines and see where they have been inconsistent. After several weeks of providing a predictable environment for their child, they can slowly begin to introduce new stimuli, just as they are slowly introducing new foods into their child's diet.

COLIC

Some extremely fussy behavior is caused by colic, in which the baby is experiencing pain, thanks to an immature digestive system. The colicky baby pulls his knees up to his chest and can howl for hours. The crying is intense and frantic and makes parents and adults extremely anxious. Colic generally goes away by the time the baby is five months old.

There is no evidence of a connection between infant colic and childhood shyness. Some families have reported that their colicky, fussy baby grew up into a hypervigilant, easily intimidated child, but it cannot be assumed that one follows another. Contact your family physician if your baby cries for hours on end and you cannot find the cause.

SOCIAL STIMULATION

The key to preparing your shy infant for a lifetime of successful social skills is to provide him with consistent, appropriate social stimulation The key word here is *appropriate*. Since too little social stimulation might lead to your child being unequipped to deal with other people, and too much social stimulation can be overwhelming in the beginning, a trial-and-error approach is necessary to create a balanced environment for your child. You will need to be observant and sympathetic; to know when to introduce new activities and people and when to allow for downtime.

Too Little Social Stimulation

It is easy to fall into daily patterns that do not provide enough social stimulation for your shy baby. In the case of a first child, the parents have so much to learn and the child needs so much that the question of adequately stimulating a child's sociability may never come up. On top of the physical attention they must give the child, mothers must adapt to their own physical changes. Postpartum depression strikes 10 to 20 percent of women. Most women suffering from postpartum depression do an adequate job caring for the immediate needs of their children, but it may be difficult for them to summon the extra effort required to provide socialization opportunities for their introverted baby.

Younger siblings may be the ones to suffer from lack of direct stimulation from parents. School-age children have their socialization needs attended to in the classroom and in the neighborhood. When parents have a lot of work to do to keep body and soul together, the needs of the youngest family member are often not considered. If the shy baby is fed, changed, and loved—and seems content to sit quietly—that is considered to be enough. Establishing a regular play group or taking the baby along to the grocery store, to the story hour at the library, or to the playground is every bit as important as signing an older sibling up for school or making sure immunization records are transferred.

Parents who leave their shy infant in the hands of a care-giver at the end of the all-too-short six weeks of maternity leave may cherish the few hours a day they have to spend with their child, and they may want her all to themselves. Mealtime and bedtime routines take up the rest of the day, and so if the child's caregiver does not take her to play with other children, the child is limited to a very isolated life. Before anyone real-izes what happens, she may develop a deep-rooted fear of other people and resist play opportunities.

Too Much Social Stimulation

Too much social stimulation creates as many problems as too little. Most babies and toddlers who experience too much so-cial stimulation do so in a crowded day care situation, or in a setting that does not have adequate adult supervision.

The first sign that a shy child is overwhelmed by social stimulation will often be fussiness. Something doesn't feel right, and he cannot tell you why. He may suck his thumb for comfort, lie down and cover his head, or lash out angrily at the person nearest him. If that doesn't bring him the comfort and reassurance he wants, he may break down into a full-blown tantrum. He may grow to dread the place where he feels overwhelmed and put up a fuss whenever it is time to go there.

When shy children are overstimulated, they feel trapped—surrounded by noise and faces, unable to make meaningful contact with anyone. Other children may be sitting too close. There is no sense of structure. The introverted child feels at the mercy of others and cannot develop social skills. Babies surrounded by too much social stimulation often sleep in brief intervals with no consistent pattern as a defense against the high activity level around them. It is the same way many adults feel in an overcrowded subway. Would you recommend a busy subway platform as a place to develop new relationships for a shy adult?

Appropriate Social Stimulation

Shy children need to be exposed to other children in play situations from the time they are infants. When a timid child spends time with other children, she learns crucial social skills that last a lifetime. When you look at two toddlers playing in the same room, they may not even seem to notice each other. They may be playing with different toys in different corners of the room. But you can be sure that each is keeping tabs on what the other is doing. These initial encounters are crucial, though there seems to be little socialization going on.

When toddlers play, they often do come together to stack blocks, imitate each other, or encroach on each other's territory and try to take toys away. Whatever they are doing, they are also learning how to share, cooperate, ask for something, stand up for themselves, value their contributions, and appreciate another person. This kind of appropriate social stimulation is the middle ground you must seek for your shy child.

KIDS NEED KIDS

Shy children who are only exposed to adults can develop an outward pseudomaturity that sometimes causes unnecessary problems. These kids tend to have expanded vocabularies and mimic adult behavior and serious demeanor. Other adults often marvel at and praise this behavior. Some consider it cute, and it doesn't take long for a child to start to enjoy the adult attention he gets. But when this pseudoadult behavior becomes habitual to the extent that it interferes with a shy child's ability to interact with peers, it is debilitating. All children need to spend time with other kids to develop naturally and in an age-appropriate manner, but it is particularly important for shy children. You don't do your kid any favors by surrounding him with adults and encouraging grown-up mannerisms. Instead, maximize playtime and peer stimulation. He'll be a more successful adult if you let him be a child first.

If Your Child Stays at Home. Parents whose children spend the first two years of life at home with one primary caregiver must find ways to give their shy little ones the chance to play with, explore, and enjoy children the same age. If there are no close neighbors who are logical candidates, then visit your local playground or library. Many friendships have started at the central fountain of the local mall or in the children's section of a bookstore.

These chance meetings are the beginnings of relationships. Alone, they will not provide your shy child with the kind of interaction she needs. Once you've met a little friend for your child, schedule regular playtimes. Invite the child and her caregiver to your home at a time when the kids are at their best, such as mid-morning. It is best to start with one friend. If you crowd four or five two-year-olds into your family room, you'll see firsthand what too much social stimulation looks like.

Your child and her guest will play together, or play beside each other for fifteen minutes if all goes well. By the fifteen-minute mark, most young children will need to come back to their caregiver for reassurance in the form of a hug or quick cuddle; a few minutes on the lap. Do not turn away from your child or reject her, or she might not want to return to playing because she's afraid you are angry or you might leave. Limit the playtime to a half hour or forty-five minutes at first. It is much better to proceed slowly than to try to force your child into doing too much, too soon.

Playtime does not always go smoothly. It is hard to share when you are two years old. Some children may want to touch their playmate's face, or throw toys across the room for fun. Parents must walk a fine line between allowing young children to work out how to play nicely and protecting the children from harm. Make sure that the children only have safe, appropriate toys to play with, and sit so that you can keep an eye on them.

Ideally, your shy infant or toddler should spend some time around other children of the same age every day, but this can be difficult. At a minimum, arrange for play group time, or visits to a park or library to be with other kids three times a week. Consistent, structured play opportunities are going to lay a foundation for healthy social skills that will benefit your child the rest of her life.

If Your Child Goes to Day Care. According to the National Center for Education Statistics, nearly 13 million infants, toddlers, and preschool children under the age of six were in child care in 1995, and 45 percent of children under age one were in child care on a regular basis. Child care is part of childrearing in America, and parents must extend their parenting concerns about shyness to their child care situation.

When you investigate day care facilities for your young shy child, do so with an eye toward her emotional as well as physical well-being. Supervision is the key. Ask who will be the primary caregiver to your child and observe that person. Be sure to observe the primary caregiver's support staff as well. Make sure that caregivers keep the children in their charge safe, occupied, and engaged. See if the facility keeps children of different ages separate. It is not safe or appropriate for an eighteen-month-old to spend all his time with five-year-olds.

Ideally, a child care arrangement will provide children with a consistent pattern of stimulation that sets good examples of interaction, problem solving, and social exchanges. A well-trained child care provider will also teach children how to transition from one social setting to another by explaining what will happen in a short time, helping children to conclude the first activity (putting away toys, saying thank you), anticipate the next activity, and then move to it.

Once your shy infant or toddler begins day care, be sure to observe her behavior. It is normal for a child to cry when she separates from her parent, but if she pitches full-blown fits every day for months, treat that as a red flag. Arrange to observe her at the day care without her being aware of your presence. If she is not receiving the right kind and amount of loving attention from adults, and does not have the chance to interact with children her age, then find another day care situation immediately.

SETTING A GOOD EXAMPLE IN SOCIAL SITUATIONS

Max's father was flabbergasted when told he demonstrated shy behavior to his little boy. This man was a high-level executive, known for strong people skills. All day he worked face-to-face with people, never flinching from interpersonal contact. In fact, he thrived on the interactions of the workplace. But when he came home from the office, he was exhausted. He didn't want to talk to anyone other than his wife and children. He let the answering machine take his phone calls, and he avoided neighborhood gatherings. Sometimes just being around his family was too much, and he retreated to the den and locked the door.

Max never saw his father as a skilled executive whom people sought out. He only saw the at-home version of dad; the man who shied away from all social contact. His father modeled behavior that said running to your room to avoid people was a good thing to do.

The maxim "Do as I say, not as I do" has gone the way of the Model T. We now know that children learn behavior by watching their parents. This observation began as soon as your child opened his eyes. If you were planning on waiting to improve your own social skills until your child could talk or was old enough to go to school, you'll be too late. Children take in information long before they can talk about it. When what you say contradicts what you do, your shy child will model his behavior on the way that you act and ignore your advice.

If you are concerned that your child is developing a degree of shyness that will interfere with his ability to make friends and feel comfortable in groups, you need to examine your own behavior as well as his. How does your child see you interact with other people?

Parents who are shy themselves face the greatest struggle. They may prefer to limit social contact, but they know first-hand what a price their children will pay if they can't bring themselves to be more outgoing. Shy parents can find that they are willing to face their shyness issues for the first time if it means helping their children develop better social skills than they have.

STRANGER AND SEPARATION ANXIETY

The two most common types of fear in the first two years of life are stranger and separation anxiety. These are normal responses to development and usually fade as a child matures if parents react appropriately. However, it can be quite upsetting when a usually cheerful child turns into one who cries hysterically whenever his mother walks out of the room, or if a checkout clerk smiles at him.

For the first six months of life, most babies respond to anyone who looks at them. Stranger anxiety normally begins around nine months, though it may start earlier. By then a baby realizes that she has primary caregivers and has matured enough to recognize it when that person goes away. The presence of a stranger seems to trigger the fear in some children that the stranger is there to replace the caregiver, and that the caregiver could leave the child alone with the stranger. Stranger anxiety usually begins to fade sometime after a baby's first birthday, especially if the child has had a lot of experience with parents and caregivers going away and always coming back. Temperamentally shy children, however, may remain wary of strangers throughout childhood.

There are a few things you can do if your child doesn't show any signs of outgrowing this fear of strangers:

- Hold your child with love and acceptance when he is scared.

- Talk to the stranger while you are holding him, keeping your body and voice relaxed.

- Try to limit the number of strangers that your child comes in contact with for a few weeks.

- Pick a person you may know distantly, such as a bank teller, librarian, or store clerk, and concentrate on exposing your child to that person every other day.

- Make meetings with strangers brief, upbeat, and friendly. The goal is to expose your child to a consistent, structured, safe method of greeting a new person. He will eventually feel safer, and grow confident in his own skills at coping with new people.

Separation anxiety usually develops along with your child's motor skills. As she learns how to crawl and walk—to move away from you—she grows to fear being away from you. Children in the middle of a separation anxiety phase may follow a parent from room to room, have a hard time falling asleep at night, and, of course, scream bloody murder when the parent has to leave them.

If your child seems to show an unusual degree of separation anxiety, try to step back and analyze the behavior. Does he scream every time you are out of sight—or when you leave him with someone else? Does he become anxious even when you just *seem* about to leave? Are there particular times of day when he reacts more strongly than others?

Remember that some separation anxiety is normal at certain stages of a child's development. However, you can make sure that you are taking steps to avoid aggravating the condition. The most important step to take in minimizing separation anxiety is to make your child's routine consistent.

- Do you have a regular baby-sitter for your child, or is he unsure of who will take care of him from one day to the next?

- Have you done all you can to be sure your child is getting an appropriate amount of attention at day care, that the caregivers who interact with your child are the same every day, and that there is nothing for him to fear?

- Do you pick up your child at the same time every day?

CHAPTER SUMMARY

1. Good socialization skills begin at birth.

2. Twenty percent of infants will show shy tendencies such as turning away from strangers and easy overstimulation.

3. Too little social stimulation leaves shy children unprepared for school and peer relationships.

4. Too much social stimulation frustrates children and prevents them from learning how to relate to others in a healthy way.

5. Parents should seek to provide their shy infant or toddler

with playtime with peers every day if possible, three times a week at a minimum.

6. Parents should observe child care settings to ensure that appropriate socialization is encouraged.

7. Parents must provide a good role model of active social skills.

Chapter 6

AGES TWO TO FIVE—
THE PRESCHOOL YEARS

This is when the fun begins. You enter new parenting territory when your child develops language skills and is old enough to explore the world more or less on her own. You discover your child as an individual with likes, dislikes, and opinions that sometimes differ from yours.

As your child develops new skills, so must you. As she strikes out on her own, her opinions and wishes sometimes come into conflict with yours. This is the time when you establish a tone for your relationship with your child that is likely to persist throughout childhood. Will you be authoritative, permissive, or somewhere in between? When your child begins to look outside from the safety of the family setting, your task is to guide her into the wider world at a pace that is comfortable for both of you.

It is also during this preschool period that you are most likely to recognize in your child the traits of a shy person.

How he explores new places, how he interacts with new acquaintances, how he approaches day care and preschool all give you clues that you are in the presence of a shy personality.

Your shy child may have an instinct for withdrawing from social contact and new experiences and a preference for solitude and the safety of home. You can help him to find a balance between the need to withdraw and the need to explore by keeping track of how new activities affect him and by challenging him with new experiences at a rate that suits his unique sensibilities. By the time your child is ready to enter kindergarten, you will have helped him achieve the self-confidence he needs to meet that new challenge.

THE POSITIVE POWER OF PRESCHOOL

Shy children need preschool. Preschool provides a crucial socialization experience that prepares them for the environment of kindergarten and elementary school. A good preschool offers structured play, supervised free time, and playmates in situations that are hard to duplicate three times a week at home. Some parents of shy children cringe at the idea of sending their child to preschool. They know that a roomful of strangers will frighten him and cause him to want to withdraw into himself, and they fear that the experience of being abandoned there will terrify or scar him. He has a hard time relating to even one child his age; how on earth will he cope with ten or twenty?

How a shy child experiences preschool depends on several factors: 1) the training and experience of the staff, 2) the pace at which she is introduced to the new environment, and

3) her parents' reaction to the signs of stress she is likely to exhibit.

Choosing a Preschool

All children deserve the highest quality preschool, but shy children in particular need a school that respects individual personalities while providing plenty of socialization opportunities. The best way to find a good preschool is to talk to parents who have sent their children there. Be sure to spend time observing the school and teacher. Don't be afraid to ask specific questions, such as how the teacher deals with children who are afraid to talk to others, or how she handles children who are reluctant to participate in activities.

As you look for the right preschool, there are several key features that will be particularly helpful for the shy child:

- Barring unexpected events, will your child have the same teachers for two or three years?

- Will pretty much the same children share the class for two or three years?

- Is class size limited?

- Is there a teacher for every four or five children?

- Is there a place in the room where your child can go to be out of the fray? A "quiet corner" or a "reading nook"?

- Is there a structure to the day in the preschool? That is, will the activities proceed in the same predictable order every day?

- Are parents allowed to observe the classroom?

Introducing Your Child to Preschool

Parents provide a necessary buffer for shy children. When the buffer is removed, the shy child feels vulnerable and lost. The "sink or swim" method of introducing preschool works for some children, but it can also cause some shy children to sink. When it comes time to introduce your child to the preschool, do so gradually. Ask permission to bring your child to the school's playground on the weekend. Bring her in for a half hour every day the first week or two, and be prepared to stay in the room. Small steps spell success for shy children. If you introduce the preschool gradually, chances are it will become a place your child looks forward to going.

Follow Up with the Teacher

You need to stay in touch with the teacher as your child adjusts to preschool by asking what he enjoys and what she notices that causes him to withdraw. Who are the children he likes to stay next to in line? Who will he look at? What are the names of other children in the class who seem a bit quiet or calm? The more information you have about the preschool, the better equipped you are to help your child. Ideally the preschool will be set up in such a way that you can observe the class without being seen by your child.

Certain problems that the teacher may report are cause for genuine concern. If your child cries constantly every day without having been hurt by other children, then she is so upset by the experience she doesn't know what to do.

If your child is still playing alone after a month of regular attendance at the preschool, discuss the situation with the teacher. If she can reassure you that your child is happy, and that it is his preference to play alone, then you can wait another month and reassess the situation. If, however, the teacher senses that your child is unable to join other children in spite of a strong desire to do so, or that the other children are rejecting him, then you should consider whether or not to continue preschool at this time.

Some children who feel socially alienated can turn to aggression to express their feelings, pushing other children away, or lashing out and hitting them. If your child is showing any of these behaviors, it is time to step in. It may be that he cannot tolerate your absence yet.

Talk to your child's teacher and ask her to be specific about the situations that are hard for your child. Ask her what your child enjoys, or share what activities your child likes at home; she should be aware of your child's preferences. If your child likes to build, then the teacher should make sure your child gets his turn at the blocks. Once your child is comfortably settled and playing with the blocks, the teacher should ask if he wants a friend to play with him. If he says no, then she needs to respect that. The goal is to increase your child's comfort level at school. He may play alone with blocks for weeks before he is ready to play with someone else.

Follow Up with Your Child

All children have bad days at school. The way you react to your child's tears or stories of frustration can influence how she acts at school. If you become overly concerned and upset, your child may grow more afraid of the preschool or the children there. If you listen with interest and then encourage your child to brainstorm creative ways to deal with tough social situations, she can come to see occasional conflict as a normal part of interacting with others.

Pretendings

When you talk about school with your child, you can use a modified type of role-playing called "pretendings" to help her work through the types of scenarios that make her anxious. Pretendings are nothing more than reenactments of typical daily situations, which, in the context of the role-play, have fun, positive conclusions. You must keep the atmosphere light and playful during pretendings. This is important work, but if it is heavy-handed, critical, or harsh, you will do more damage than good.

When your child is rested, fed, and in a good mood, play pretend. "Let's pretend you're at school and you're playing with the blocks . . ." is a good way to begin. Get out the blocks and get on the floor with your child. You can pretend to be another child in the class, using a name of a friendly child you have heard about from the teacher, or someone your child has mentioned. Use "what if" scenarios: "What if Alex came over? What could you say?" Remember to be silly sometimes: "What if Alex flew on a dinosaur around the room and asked you if you wanted to ride with him? What if you flew to the moon?"

The goal is to get your child to think about interacting with others without feeling tense. Keep pretending sessions short and spontaneous; no more than fifteen minutes. If your child is resisting or acts bored, cut the session short.

You can also use pretending sessions to help your child identify the things about him that would make him interesting to playmates:

Tony was an athletic five-year-old who had an extremely hard time opening up to other children. His classmates had given up on him and no longer made an effort to play with him.

To help him become more sociable, his parents brainstormed with him about what he was good at—what he could do that might interest other children. Tony was very good at standing on his head, so his parents suggested that he do that during the play period at school. He wasn't sure it would have any effect, but agreed to try.

He came home extremely excited and proud of himself. When he stood on his head, the class crowded around, asking how he did that and trying it themselves. He found himself explaining a few basic things about balance, and talking easily to kids who had ignored him the day before. "I can't believe they wanted to know about standing on your head," he told his parents. Tony continued with pretendings, developing skills at home to ask someone to play, how to share toys, and, one of the hardest skills, how to ask to be included in a group.

ALONE TIME

It may seem counterintuitive to recommend solitude for shy children, but it is necessary for their development and health. Social stimulus provokes anxiety in shy children and it can be mentally exhausting. Children need time to unwind, just as adults do.

In most communities, so many opportunities for children exist that many well-meaning parents pack their children's schedules with extracurricular activities. If your shy child attends a half-day preschool program five days a week, then he has ample time in school for rich social opportunities. It is most likely that he does not need extra socialization on top of that.

Let him play alone when he gets home from school if that is what he wants to do. If he wants to play with friends, or you decide to set up a play date, then arrange for time between school and the next engagement when he can relax and be alone or just with the family. Your child will have more fun and be more successful if he has a chance to recharge his emotional batteries.

CAN I PLAY?

The neighborhood kids played in the cul-de-sac in front of little Alisha's house. There were long-running games of kickball, tag, and Wiffle ball. The cul-de-sac was sometimes covered in chalk when the kids created an entire pretend village. Alisha sat on the steps of her front porch day after day, and her mother knew that she longed to join in. But nothing would persuade her to approach the group of children.

Her mother tried everything to push her daughter into the action, all to no avail. Alisha simply did not know how to join the group. Was it fear of rejection that stopped her? Not knowing what to say?

Learning how to break into a game or group of other children playing together is very hard for shy children. Their negative social appraisal kicks in and they assume that the kids don't want them there. They may assume that if they were wanted, someone would come over and issue an invitation. In reality, of course, other children assume that if a child is sitting on the porch and not joining in, that is the child's preference.

A shy child may imagine all kinds of bad reactions if he were to put himself forward. Eventually he can convince himself that no matter what he does or says, the group will reject him. Even if your shy child is getting along well in preschool, it may be difficult for her to join in when the kids in the neighborhood get together, especially if she or the other children are more or less newcomers to the neighborhood. For one thing, neighborhood groups tend to have a larger mix of age ranges and the older children dominate, usually without much regard for the feelings of the younger children.

Kids playing kickball or tag outside typically don't have much adult supervision, so there isn't a grown-up to make sure that everyone gets a turn or feels included. And last, your preschool child may be too small, or not understand the rules of a game played by older children, and he doesn't feel comfortable showing his ignorance of the game.

Outgoing children operate with a different set of assumptions. They seem to know instinctively that if they go and stand on the edge of a group of kickball players, someone will notice them and bring them into the game. If that doesn't happen, they have no trouble asking bluntly if they can play. If they are told no, they usually don't give up easily. They ask why, or they take a different tack, suggesting ways in which they can be involved, or reminding people of other times when they welcomed kids into a game. They stick around, waiting for a chance to participate.

The issue of social persistence is one of the things that separates shy from nonshy children. When an outgoing child is rejected by a group, he tends to think that the group has lost out by being deprived of his presence; then he moves on to thinking of something else to do, or another friend he can contact. When a shy child is rejected, he takes it to heart where the pain burns long after the incident. The shy child assumes that a rejection is permanent. Because they said he couldn't play kickball once, he'll never ask again.

Even if your child screws up her courage, joins the games, and follows all the rules, the other kids may reject her. This does not have to be a disaster. Learning how to deal with rejection and the feeling of failure is important for all children, but it is particularly difficult for shy children. The trick is to turn the rejection into a teachable moment.

Strategies to Encourage Group Involvement

You can use pretending sessions to help your preschooler learn to manage her fear of asking to play. Dolls or action figures work very well. Get on the floor with your child and act out a group of dolls playing and their reactions when a new doll wants to join in. Don't limit yourself to the predictable responses. Exaggerate and be silly. Your child needs the chance to laugh about these feelings.

When you pretend play situations with your child, be sure to work with the pretending scenario of the group absolutely refusing to let the new doll join in. Introduce the idea of "pick yourself up, dust yourself off, and start all over again." Be physical: Go through the motions of picking yourself up off the floor, dusting yourself off, and finding something else to do, all the while talking out loud to yourself: "It doesn't matter that they said no to me. I'll find something else to do. I'll play with my jump rope, or I'll wash my bike. But I'm going to stay here where they can see me, and I'll ask if I can play in a little while. I'm going to stick with it until they include me in their game!"

An excellent strategy for helping a child get involved in a neighborhood group is to enlist the help of an older child. Choose someone whose family you are friendly with, or it could be your baby-sitter or your baby-sitter's sibling. Have a quiet word with an older child you trust and ask if she could make sure that your child is occasionally invited to join the fun. The other children will be much more responsive to a suggestion from one of their own than if you try to shoehorn your kid into the action.

By far the most effective strategy for getting your child to integrate into the neighborhood is to give her time to play one-on-one with neighborhood children. By observing children at play, you can usually identify which children would get on best with your child. By getting to know the parents in the neighborhood, you can set up play dates at your own house, and, over time, one or two of the children will almost certainly become good friends with your child. Then, when the whole crowd is out playing kickball or tag, it will be much easier for your child to approach the group knowing there are one or two children who know her and accept her.

WHEN YOU HEAR YOUR HEART BREAKING

Watching your child skirt the edge of a group and give up in frustration can be agonizing—for you! You know what the scene looks like: A group of children plays happily together, digging in a sandbox, riding bikes in a driveway, or chasing bubbles in the backyard. Your child is not smiling, or laughing, or giggling with the others. Your child stands off to the side, watching the other children, biting her lip, looking away when any other child approaches her. Nothing you say or do will make your child join in the fun.

Few things hurt as much as watching your child in pain. Your emotions are a tangle of guilt, fear, and anxiety. Why can't he just join in? Is there something wrong with him? Have you been a bad parent? How is he ever going to survive school?

Do not give in to your fears. The worst thing you can do is to allow your own pain to overwhelm you because your child will pick up on it instantly. As hard as it seems, your remaining objective and calm is just what your child needs, even when he runs to you with tears in his eyes.

You can be empathetic, but do not commiserate. If you try to soothe the hurt by distracting him with promises of candy, ice cream, trips, and fun for just the two of you, you do not solve his problem. Rather, you paper over it and put yourself in the position of his savior. If this way of dealing with his hurts becomes habitual, it can only emphasize his sense of his own inadequacy in dealing with social situations. You can help him, but you need to avoid letting him become dependent on you.

You can't expect your child to learn how to toughen up his feelings if you melt every time he feels awkward. This is one time when you should lead with your head, not your heart.

MANIPULATION

With children, it is sometimes necessary to take a hard look at their behavior and distinguish between their honest reactions to situations and their deliberate attempts to manipulate you. All children—shy or not—will try to manipulate their parents from time to time. If your child learns that you give in to his desires when he shows shy behaviors, he may try to use them to get what he wants.

There are physiological and behavioral differences you will see between genuine shy behavior and pretend shyness. If your child is truly feeling anxious, you will see it in his body. He will show standard stress reactions such as rapid, shallow breathing, sweating on his face, palms, and under his arms, and his heart will beat quickly. He will show real avoidance behavior and will withdraw. If he is truly in distress, he won't negotiate. Shy children usually don't whine; instead, they act afraid. A genuine fear reaction is very hard to fake.

However, if you have a shy child you feel is trying to manipulate you, it is better to respond conservatively, with care and love, than it is to confront him. Be sure to examine the situation that seems to be causing the manipulative behavior and take the entire day in context. Remember that establishing and maintaining a strong relationship with your child is the best way to help him develop self-confidence.

PARENTAL MODELING

We don't realize how much our children watch us. Every minute we are together, they are learning. This can be good news when our behavior is what we want our children to emulate. But our own habits are more often less than perfect.

You must be aware of your own behavior before you can expect your child to improve his. If a father swipes French fries from his wife's plate without asking permission, he is not following the rules about sharing he expects from his own children. If he then punishes his child for taking without asking, the child may be confused or lose respect for his father's teachings.

It is hard for adults to observe their own behavior objectively because so much of it is unconscious habit. Even when they are concerned about their children's actions, parents have a hard time seeing how their actions influence their child. A group of parents who assembled for a workshop on shyness in children provided a classic example. The parents cautiously entered the room, averting their eyes, staying to the edges of the room, and not talking to anyone they didn't know. No one would enter the center of the room, or even sit down in a chair. They were waiting and observing, just like the shy children who were watching them, learning how to interact in a group.

Talking Out Loud

You can begin to show your shy child good assertive problem-solving skills by talking more. Let him know what you are thinking. If you are in a department store and you can't find the umbrellas, but you are a little unsure of asking for help, then say to your child, "I'm nervous, and I wish I didn't have to talk to a store clerk, but I'm going to ask that one to help me."

This is called "spontaneous verbal compensation," and it is a form of verbalizing your self-talk. It may astonish your child the first few times you try it. He may be shocked to learn, first, that other people engage in self-talk and, second, that you feel anxious and unsure of yourself sometimes. Admitting these feelings is a sign of strength, not an admission of weakness. You are teaching the most important secret about courage: that it is the management of fear, not the absence of it.

When you are letting your child into this part of your emotions, be sure to do it in real time, not after the fact. Nothing is more boring to a little kid than to listen to a parent drone on about something that is over: "Did you see what Daddy did back there? Did you see how Daddy asked for directions?" Well, frankly, no; your child probably wasn't paying attention. But if you keep him engaged by explaining what you are thinking and why you are doing something, he will feel involved and will learn the lesson you want to share.

Your child also learns by watching you interact with other children. If the presence of a five-year-old stranger makes you tongue-tied and self-conscious, then it is unlikely that your shy child will strike up a conversation with the kid. Say hello to the children that you meet in the hall of preschool or at the park. Keep your language and expression friendly, but avoid talking down to the child. Whatever you do, don't torture your child with well-meaning but hurtful phrases such as, "See I talked to the little boy—it wasn't so hard. Why can't you do that?" Provide a good example and allow your child the time and space he needs to grow.

Positive Assertiveness

Dealing with interpersonal conflict is uncomfortable for many of us, not just the shy. However, showing your child how you handle everyday uncomfortable situations can go a long way toward increasing her own comfort level when asking for things or standing her ground.

If you know you are going to stop by the dry cleaner to complain that they did not remove a stain properly, be sure to bring along your preschooler. (Do not run this errand when she's tired and hungry—that's a recipe for disaster. Bring her when she is fresh, rested, and happy.) The conversation you have with the dry cleaner in which you calmly explain the situation and ask that they fix the problem will be instructive and useful for your child.

Calling In Reinforcements

If you know that you don't always set the best example for your shy child, then call in reinforcements. Arrange to have your child spend time with a relative or close friend who is outgoing, positive, and constructive. The adult can take your child shopping, or to places where together they can interact with other children. Time spent with a favorite "aunt" or "uncle" like this can provide a tremendous boon to your child. She will learn a different model of social interaction, and may be a bit more relaxed and willing to engage other children. One note of caution: Make sure that the person you choose is someone you know very well, and is a safe person who would never harm your child.

GETTING READY FOR BIG-KID SCHOOL

The transition from home to school is one of the most difficult ones your child will ever make. That is part of the significance of a positive preschool experience. Preschool allows your child to adjust to being away from the home environment and the care of parents and to the sometimes unsettling sensations associated with a room of children his age.

As your child approaches five years old, you will want to start drawing pictures of elementary school if your child doesn't bring up the subject on her own. You should draw the bus, or a picture of your child walking; represent how your child will get to school. Take cues from your conversations with your child and use the drawing sessions as a fun way to help her anticipate what "big-kid school" will be like.

There are a number of other things you can do to prepare your child for the transition to kindergarten, whether he has attended preschool or not. Take your child to visit the elementary school regularly. If he has an older sibling at the school, then bring him along every time you go to school. If you are dropping off cupcakes for a birthday party, or picking up forms at the nurse's office, bring the shy younger sibling to school every chance you get. It may seem inconvenient, and you might be tempted to leave the little one with a baby-sitter or neighbor, but a little inconvenience now will pay off in the long run.

Every time your shy child has a positive experience in the elementary school, he is building up an account of good feelings that he will draw from if kindergarten overwhelms him. The goal is to make elementary school a familiar and friendly place. Remember that settings have a huge influence on shy children. If he knows where the bathrooms are, and the librarians and principal know his face and name, then he will approach big-kid school with confidence and enthusiasm.

Even if you don't have an older child already attending the elementary school, you are still welcome there. Take your shy child to the playground on the weekends or after school is dismissed. Go to the office and ask for a calendar of events. Most elementary schools have several events that are open to the community. When you attend, make sure to tour the school, showing your shy child the classrooms, bathrooms, and cafeteria. Meet with the principal and ask if you can bring

your child in to visit a kindergarten class before the end of the
school year. Every time your shy child visits the school, he becomes more comfortable in it and improves his chances of
having a great time in kindergarten.

CHAPTER SUMMARY

1. Preschool-aged children are wonderful and fun to be
   around. They can share with you what they see and think
   of the world with their increased language and observational skills.

2. Preschool-aged children can learn a great deal about social interaction at a well-supervised preschool.

3. Parents should stay in close touch with teachers and observe their shy child at preschool to understand the child's
   problems.

4. Parents can use pretendings to help their child learn how
   to work through anxiety-producing situations.

5. Parents who feel upset about their child's exclusion from
   play groups must react with their heads, not their hearts.

6. Parents must be sure to model excellent socialization behaviors in front of their children.

7. Shy parents can use loving, outgoing adult friends to show
   their children good examples of social skills.

8. Familiarize your child with his elementary school at a
   young age by visiting the playground and spending time
   in the school itself.

Chapter 7

THE ELEMENTARY SCHOOL YEARS

Parents who have worked hard to help their shy child during the preschool years may be dismayed to find a whole new set of challenges when the child begins elementary school. The intimate settings of home and preschool give way to a much larger social and educational environment. Friends go off to different schools, and your child faces the prospect of making new friends. The preschool teacher who had finally earned your child's confidence is replaced by a teacher he does not know, and who knows nothing about him.

As more dimensions are added to your child's life, suddenly he has much more to think about than ever before: home, school, friends, neighborhood, sports teams, and outside activities. At the same time the emotional development your child is going through can sometimes mean that he feels pain or rejection more acutely, or that his social anxiety is heightened. But his expanded horizons give him more opportunities to succeed, and his maturity gives him new tools to work with.

The constant social interactions of elementary school can seem overwhelming to your child. On the other hand, the opportunities for growth are plentiful during these socially and developmentally rich years. If you are actively working with your child to help him cope with anxious feelings and nurture his self-confidence, you will find plenty of chances for your child to test his fledgling social skills.

DEVELOPMENTAL CHANGES

Around age six the typical child begins to develop a more complete sense of herself as an individual outside of her family unit. She evaluates herself in relation to others and recognizes her separateness. Whether or not she is shy, her internal dialogue begins to include statements such as, "I am the kind of person who likes music" or "I am the kind of person who likes to read a lot," or negative messages such as, "I am the kind of person that nobody wants to be around."

Parents can help children in this phase by clarifying preferences aloud. "Are you the kind of person who enjoys cats?" "What kind of person likes to help?" or "What about the color red?" Such questions, made without a hint of judgment, let the child explore her individuality, recognizing its legitimacy and value.

By the same token, children recognize that they share personality traits with some children and not with others. "I am the kind of person who likes cats, but John likes dogs better. Richard also likes cats." The ability to find common ground with others is based on the self-awareness of personal preferences and the awareness that others have preferences too. Finding common ground is often the basis of friendship. Accepting the differences of others is the basis of cooperation, tolerance, and play.

During the elementary years the concept of "popularity" enters into the picture. Children acquire the sense of who is popular and who is not. They become keenly aware of the limits of their friends and themselves. Children who have played together for years may lose interest in each other, or may deliberately avoid each other as they see where their friends fall on the popularity scale. Shy children may find themselves abandoned by a special friend who suddenly considers the shy child a liability, someone who does not seek favorable attention.

As social relationships become more complex, those children who excel at social skills tend to be the most popular. Shy children, who may be more interesting or empathetic, are often left behind. From an adult's perspective, the concept of popularity may seem trivial and superficial. But like it or not, it is important to realize that for most children the issue can be all-consuming.

Shy children respond to the notion of popularity in different ways. They may have a keen desire to be popular, and that desire may lead to despair when their social skills don't measure up. Some reject the whole idea of popularity and develop pride in being different. They deliberately set themselves apart from the "popular crowd" and often make close friendships with others who see themselves as separate. While more naturally outgoing children tend to blame others for their lack of popularity, some shy children blame themselves and dwell on their social failures. As the parent of a shy child, you will need to become sensitive to the way your child is handling social pressure during the elementary years and to approach the issue with compassion and understanding.

SCHOOL DAYS

Most children enter elementary school with trepidation. Outgoing children survey the expanded social environment with a sense of excitement that usually overrides the awkwardness of the situation. This is a new opportunity for them to show their stuff and to join with others. If a child is fundamentally an extrovert, he draws energy from other people: The more people, the more energy. The child who enjoys attention and knows how to use it sees the new teacher as a new world to master. He starts to impress the teacher right away with whatever it is he recognizes as his particular gifts or strengths.

The shy child, being focused internally, often experiences other people as draining his energy, and he may come home from school feeling extremely tired. With his newly developing sense of himself, he may feel insecure about his differences, may be hyperaware of his separateness, and may feel that he doesn't fit in anywhere in this new environment. If his initial impression is that school is a place where he can't succeed socially, he may begin to use his intellectual skills to find ways to avoid having any attention drawn to him. It is possible for a child to devote almost all his coping skills to accomplishing this disappearing act.

Two weeks into her son Alex's first year in elementary school, his mother, Jane, watched through the chain-link fence. Alex was swinging aimlessly around the flagpole, while other children swirled around him, laughing and engaged with each other. He didn't seem upset, embarrassed, or even aware that other children were present. But Jane knew he was feeling all those emotions. When a boy his age ran up to Alex and invited him to play, Alex shook his head silently. The boy walked away.

When she waved to her son, Alex ran over. He was smiling, not seeming at all distressed or anxious. "How was your day?" she asked. "Fun," he answered, sounding sincere. "What did you do?" "Oh, nothing."

The bell rang, and Alex lined up to go inside. He looked back to make sure she was watching. Meanwhile, the friendly boy who had invited him to play approached Jane with a helpful explanation, "That's Alex. He doesn't talk!"

Elementary school is a thoroughly social environment, and it necessarily takes place out of a parent's range. You may often feel like Jane; forced to watch a scenario unfold that seems awkward for your child, but because you cannot be there with him, you feel powerless to help. It may feel like your shy elementary school child will be miserable forever. Do not despair. By understanding how your child perceives school situations and using the rolls of daily discussion and role-playing, your child can become comfortable, confident, and in control. There are also steps you can take to be a part of your child's initiation into elementary school.

The School Building

For a small child, the physical surroundings of a new school can seem overwhelming. Huge buildings may be a source of anxiety for the shy child because he does not know how to ask for help if he gets lost. One teacher told the story of frantically searching for a first grader who never made it back from music class on the third day of school. The principal found him curled up in a cubby, trying to be brave, but not daring to ask any of the several people who walked by without noticing him how to get back to his first-grade classroom.

Then there was the case of the boy who entered a new school in second grade. He asked to go to the bathroom and was gone much too long. The teacher went in, only to find that the boy could not get the stall unlocked, and there was not enough room to crawl under the door. Many children had come into the bathroom during the time he was locked in, but he did not ask for help. He was, of course, in tears of shame and fear by the time the teacher coaxed him out.

If you know your child is shy, then you can anticipate such situations by going with her into any new building she will have to learn to negotiate and showing her around. You can playfully look for bathrooms, check how locks work, make her familiar with hallways, and, most important, show her the route to the office where she is sure to be noticed if she is lost. As you walk the hallways, look for other significant adults, the cafeteria helpers, and custodian, the librarian, and help your child make a connection with as many as possible.

Whether your child is entering kindergarten or first grade or starting a new school as an older elementary student, taking the time to go with him to the school before it starts is one of the most helpful tasks you can accomplish. The goal is to give your child a sense of ownership over the environment. Find as many ways as you can to say to your child, "This is *your* school."

Show your child how to get from one important place to the next. Say to your child, "This is where I'll drop you off in the mornings (or where the bus will stop). Let's see how you get to your class from here." Be as positive about how convenient the route is.

Early Teacher Contact

If possible, contact the school in the spring and arrange to talk with the teacher who will have your child in the fall. Some districts do not make room assignments until the end of summer; don't be discouraged if you are asked to call back later. When you talk to the teacher, ask if you can stop by a few days before school starts to help acquaint your child with the building and her classroom.

In your advance call to the teacher, you might ask if she has already assigned desks. Letting your child see and sit in her own chair or desk is an extraordinary benefit. An outgoing child who enters a strange classroom with the task of looking for the desk with her name on it finds the whole thing enormously exciting, like an Easter egg hunt. The shy child, on the other hand, can be concerned about making a mistake. She might have worried on the way to school that there will be no desk for her. She might have built up any number of worries that simply seeing the desk in advance will alleviate.

If you can arrange it, go to the classroom at a time when the teacher is there. Shy children do best in initial one-on-one encounters, especially with adults. If you are shy, you might have a hard time arranging this meeting; you might feel you are imposing on the teacher's time. Don't worry; that's what he's there for. An astute teacher will recognize your child's shy personality and will, you hope, go out of his way to help her through the first days.

Model appropriate communication with the teacher. Ask frankly about the location of the bathroom, for example, and ask what the policy is on going there during the school day. If you are not shy, you will be surprised to learn the number of children who spend miserable hours not knowing how to ask this simple question. Of course, you can assume the teacher will go over such procedures on the first day of school, but it is valuable for your child to hear you ask, to know that the teacher will respond kindly. And remember that your child will likely be tuning in to an enormous amount of stimuli on that first day, finding it difficult to concentrate on what the teacher says.

Some teachers are very good at asking direct questions of children and waiting patiently for them to answer while pretending that a parent is not standing by. Others will let you answer for your child if you do it. Here is another area where you must be sensitive. Insisting that a child answer a strange and important adult when he seems, to all appearances, to be melting from embarrassment is not productive. Answering every question for him, though, might set a bad precedent. If you see that he simply cannot answer direct questions from the teacher, then it is probably all right to intervene. Give him a little time, though. He might just be mustering his courage. (See "The Daily Discussion for Elementary School," p. 172, for ideas for practicing questions and answers at home.)

From the classroom, investigate routes to the cafeteria, the office, the bus or car pool waiting area. Keep your eyes peeled for potential problem areas. Introduce yourself and your child to all friendly looking adults along the way: the custodian and cafeteria workers, the principal, the guidance counselor, the school secretary. Remember that besides adding to the number of friendly faces she will recognize during the first week of school, you are constantly modeling for your child how one goes about making introductions and starting conversations.

Be frank with your child about his difficulty in asking for help. You can explore this during your daily discussions. If there is a situation from the recent past that you can use as an example, say to your child, "Do you remember when you couldn't find me that day in the grocery store, and I told you which people you could ask next time? I know you are the kind of person who has a hard time asking for directions, but just remember that when you don't know what to do, you can go to the office, and Mrs. Sewell or Mr. Sullivan will know just what to do." Also, plan for the exceptions, the unexpected events. What if your child gets to school early and finds the classroom door locked? Where will he go for help?

If the teacher or school secretary has a list of your child's classmates, check to see which children live nearby and which will ride the same bus. If any of the children are already acquaintances with your child, it will be worth carpooling with their parents for the first few days of school so that your child can enter the classroom with his friends. Try to arrange to meet some parents and children who will be in your child's class. This is especially important if your child is new to the school or one who knows no one in the class. Even if your shy child cannot be counted upon to interact with a new child in such a contrived situation, you can meet the parents, model good conversational skills, and give your child a chance to study at least a few of the other students. Most other parents will be happy when you initiate this kind of late-summer contact. You can arrange to meet in a park or at a fast-food restaurant where the children can be active together without either one having to play host.

FIRST DAYS

- Even if your child is going to ride the bus to school, it is a good idea to do what you can to arrange to drive him to school on the first day.

- Be sensitive to what your child needs. Some children want their parents to walk into the classroom; others are mortified at the thought. Most kindergartners and first graders do not object to their parents' presence, and there will probably be quite a few parents doing the same thing. An older child entering a new school is more likely to resist your accompanying him to the classroom.

- Whether you mingle with other parents in the classroom or at the drop-off place, model relaxed social behavior. Walking around and greeting other parents is a way to be close to your child without being *too* close. Talk to other children; reintroduce yourself and your child to the teacher.

- Be sensitive to your child's cues. Try to assess how much he needs you and how much he can handle on his own. You can evaluate his real thinking on the subject during your daily discussions.

- If you drive your child to school, observe who she goes to after she gets out of the car. It might be painful for you to see that, during the first weeks or months, she hangs back from any social interaction. At home, rehearse potential social situations during the time before school begins.

- When you are together in the evenings during this first week, frame your questions carefully. If your child has not been able to connect yet, you do not want to give the impression that there is something wrong. Remember that shy children are notorious watchers. They wait to find a niche they can fill in the social scene. (Your child *might* be miserable before and after school and during recess, or he *might* be enjoying figuring out the complex relationships unfolding before him.) Ask open-ended questions that take into account this tendency to watch.

TEACHERS

On the day before parent-teacher conferences at Rachel's school, Rachel's mother asked her what issues to raise with the teacher. She knew how to ask questions so Rachel would reveal something of her inner world. A yes-or-no question such as, "Do you like your teacher?" would elicit very little information. Even a more specific question, "What is your teacher like?" usually got the unsatisfactory answer, "She's nice."

Rachel's mom asked, "What is the best thing about your teacher?" Rachel answered, "She ends the class twenty minutes early every day and reads us a story." Then Mom asked, "What is the worst thing about your teacher?" The answer told her what she needed to talk to the teacher about. "Well," said Rachel, "she doesn't treat everybody the same." Mom prodded. "Well, she changed the seats and I'm in the back, and she never calls on me. And when she checks homework, she just looks at mine for a second, but when she looks at other people's, she tells them how good it is." When Rachel named the kids who had been put in the front of the class, her mother knew that they were the ones who needed the most help academically, and the ones who were the most likely to be discipline problems.

During the conference with Rachel's teacher, her mother tactfully brought up the issue of Rachel's feeling that the teacher gave her little praise. As you might expect, the teacher was surprised to find out that Rachel wanted that kind of attention. In fact, the teacher said, "I think of Rachel as wholly self-contained and competent. Other students clearly need constant affirmation, but Rachel seems to get along fine without it."

Teachers assume that most school-age children will make their needs known, but the shy child may be unable to express her needs due to fear of shame, embarrassment, or being judged.

Another reason the shy child has difficulty entering the larger world of elementary school is that, in classes that sometimes hold as many as twenty-five to thirty-five students, a child who is competent at her schoolwork and shows no behavioral problems may be overlooked by the teacher. Remember that, though the child seems to be doing everything in her power to avoid attracting attention, she may at the same time be spending an inordinate amount of interior time wishing the teacher would recognize her abilities.

It is tempting to fault the teacher for not realizing that *all* children need positive feedback. But if your own child has perfected a disappearing act, then you can appreciate the word the teacher used to describe Rachel: *self-contained*. It was meant as a compliment. Rachel was quite successful at convincing her teacher that she didn't need attention. Meanwhile, the great paradox of the shy child's life was at work: She dreaded being the center of attention, but she wanted more than anything for that teacher to notice her.

If the squeaky wheel gets the grease, then the wheel that doesn't squeak obviously doesn't need any grease. That's the message your child may impart to teachers who are not alert to the ways of the shy child. It becomes part of your job to help her learn appropriate ways to get the grease if she wants it.

Teachers As Observers

A better way to use teachers, though, is to realize that most are excellent observers of behavior, and they accumulate a wealth of information just by watching children every day. When you plan a conversation with your child's teacher, think of it as more of a fact-*finding* mission than a fact-*giving* mission. If your child is saying little but doing his work, the teacher is not likely to express concern on account of his silence. You may have to ask direct questions about his social interactions and his willingness to participate in class activities. The feedback can help you structure your daily discussions with your child and set goals.

It is not necessarily a good idea to involve teachers in active therapies for a shy child. However, if you know your child is longing for attention and not getting it, it does not hurt to let the teacher know that directing praise toward your child and calling on him more often will mean more to him than she realizes.

If you are actively working with your child on her shyness—that is, if you are working with her to set daily goals—you can certainly let the teacher know what they are. For example, suppose in your conversations with your child, she has expressed an interest in striking up a friendship with a certain classmate. You have been suggesting ways for her to do that and have been following her progress by gently inquiring each day. By cluing the teacher in, you can ask her to observe what progress your child makes and to be generous in providing time for friendship building of this type. If she's willing, she might even find ways to put the two children together in low-pressure situations—cleaning paintbrushes together, for example—where it will be easier for your child to practice her skills. Teachers can be tremendous reinforcers in this way.

You should encourage your child to talk with his teacher when there is something he doesn't understand about rules or grades or any aspect of school life. When your child seems confused about the teacher's decisions, that presents an excellent opportunity to write a script with him that he can use to get more information from the teacher.

Often a shy child hopes with all his heart that by describing a problem to you, you will go to the teacher and get the problem straightened out. Of course, there will be times when this kind of intervention is necessary. But an obvious goal for the shy child is to learn to fight his own battles. Rehearsals during daily discussions that include you playing the part of the teacher can be fun while building your child's communication skills.

A NOTE ABOUT SIBLINGS

An older sibling can help make the early weeks of school bearable for the shy child. Meeting an older sibling can provide breaks in the day when the shy child can relax. If they meet on the playground or in the cafeteria, and if the older child openly brings the younger into *her* circle of friends, then the younger can enjoy some respite from the fear or not fitting in. Even if they do not physically interact, an older, more outgoing sibling can be a reassuring sight and can also model good friendship-building skills for the shy child.

The sibling relationship in school can be a mixed blessing, however. If your younger and older children have the same recess period, and the younger always makes a beeline for the older's social group, it can slow her progress in her own social group. Sometimes an older sibling's friends adopt the younger as a kind of mascot, making the shy child feel welcome. Their affection might be genuine, but there are many pitfalls to this kind of reliance on an older group.

When you have an opportunity to speak with your child's teacher, be sure to ask about playground activity. If either the younger or the older child's teacher has noticed that your shy child has developed a dependency on the older child's friends to get through recess period, then you may need to enlist the help of the teachers to break the pattern. Although this kind of sibling relationship is a sign of tolerance and love for one another, it is imperative that the younger child make her own relationships with friends her own age. She need not give up her sister's friends, but she will not be able to depend on them for long.

THE DAILY DISCUSSION FOR ELEMENTARY SCHOOL

The elementary school years are ideal for engaging your shy child in the daily discussion. At this age, children are old enough to understand the concept of shyness and to know that they may wish to overcome it. They are amazingly adept at constructing hypothetical scenarios, and most are perfectly capable of imagining what each person in the scenario will do in a given situation. Before age six, children are usually not able to grasp the long-term goal of managing shyness, and later, during their adolescence, they are often unwilling to participate in rehearsal and role-playing. Between the ages of six and eleven or twelve, though, daily discussion, rehearsing, and role-playing can be terrific fun and extremely productive.

The first goal of the daily discussion is to give your child an outlet both for hashing out the events of the day and for learning to evaluate his self-talk. Remember that shy children at this age often have a very hard time even identifying their feelings, let alone expressing them, and they usually do not tune in to their own self-talk unless you help. The daily discussion is aimed at allowing you to discover what your child is *thinking*, which is much easier than discovering what he is feeling. Inevitably, feelings will come out, and that is all to the good. A child's play is linked directly to their thinking. Keep in mind that your child's *thoughts* are the starting points for every discussion.

Shy children have marvelously complex self-talk, and teaching them to listen to it and test it for positive or negative qualities is a long-term goal for all parents. If you have already set a pattern for daily discussions before your child reaches the elementary school years, you already know that the abundance of new information your child is processing as she enters school must be sorted through one bit at a time. If you are beginning now to work on shyness with your child, you will need to remind yourself frequently that you and your child are embarking on a journey together that will be accomplished in tiny steps over a long period of time. You will both find rich rewards all along the way, but there will be periods when it seems as though you are standing still. Patience is the key.

One way parents unwittingly stop their children from talking openly during the daily discussion is to rely on yes-or-no questions. Asking open-ended questions that imply no judgment is crucial to keeping the discussion going. Some examples of open-ended questions are:

- *What did you learn that you'd never learned before?* (Not: Did you learn anything new?)

- *What talking did you do today?* (Not: Who did you talk with today? *or* Did you talk today?)

- *What happened during math (or recess, or lunch) today?* (Not: What did you do at school today?)

- *What did you think when the teacher yelled at Nathan?* (Not: Were you afraid? *or* Did you think she would yell at you too?)

If you set up the rules of the daily discussion according to the plan in Part I, your child will soon believe that he can say anything without fear of judgment or shame. You can consistently reinforce this trust by keeping your tone of voice, facial expression, and body language all neutral, and by the nature of the questions you ask.

Identifying and Stopping Negative Self-Talk

The first goal in holding daily discussions with your child is to help her identify negative self-talk, to practice stopping negative thoughts, and to replace them with neutral or positive ones. After your child has shared her thoughts about what happened in the day, and the two of you have identified which thoughts are negative or painful, then you can tag them so that if they come up on the next day, your child will remember to try to stop them. (This is where creating a visual prop, such as an index card with the key words on it, will help the child remember.) For example:

You are sitting with your nine-year-old, and one of the things she has told you is that the two girls who sit across from her in class are always whispering together. They laugh a lot, and your child is sure they are talking about her. By asking a few judicious questions, you realize that, in fact, these two girls really may have made your daughter the object of their scorn. You ask your child what she thinks about when this happens. She might say something such as, "I think there must be something wrong with me," or "I think they don't like me." These might escalate into more general statements, "Nobody likes me," or "I think I'm weird."

After her thoughts on the subject of the unpleasant girls are on the table, your child can begin to look more closely at them. Write her statements down on index cards and go through them together. You can help by asking, "Which of those thoughts seem to be negative self-talk?" Your challenge as the parent is to learn how to raise this question without implying that your child should never have negative thoughts. It is natural for her to have these thoughts; the trust you establish with your child comes from the notion that you are on the same team, and your mutual goal is to accept that negative self-talk is normal. At the same time, you are trying to teach your child that it is in her best interest to try to alter it.

Once the negative thoughts are identified, you can remind your child to watch for these phrases the next day. You remind her to say to herself, "Stop," or "Clear," or to imagine a stop sign. Another technique is to tell your child to consider the negative thought as a door leading to a place where she is not allowed to go because it is harmful to her. When a negative thought, such as "Nobody likes me," comes up, she says to herself immediately, "Can't go there." She can visualize herself turning away from the door and heading for another, more positive door.

Negative self-talk can be replaced by neutral or positive self-statements. You and your child can brainstorm possible alternative thoughts during the daily discussion. Then she will have them at her fingertips the next time she thinks negatively about herself. Possible alternatives to the thoughts she has about herself when the other girls are mean include:

- *I think they don't like me.* (Stop! They don't know me. People who know me like me. *Or*, Amanda likes me; she's my best friend.)

- *Nobody likes me.* (Stop! I know three people who like me. *Or*, I am a fun and likable person.)

- *I think I'm weird.* (Stop! It is weird to make fun of people. I don't make fun of people. *Or*, I like being different from other people.)

Neutral self-statements can be as simple as "I am okay" or "It will be okay." The purpose of the exercise is for the child to be able to *identify* negative self-talk as soon as it occurs, to *stop* the negative thought, and to *replace* it rather than dwell on it. Remember that sometimes it takes saying Stop! more than once to halt the negative thought and replace it. Every time you get a negative thought stopped, your control increases.

Anticipating the Unexpected

The daily discussions can provide time to talk about unexpected events that might happen in the life of an elementary school child, and to plan for how to handle them. For example, suppose you drop your child off at school every day on your way to work. Using your imagination, you can guess at some things that might go wrong. What if, for example, you drop your child off a little early one day, and he finds the school door locked and no other kids around. What will he do? It may seem odd to put fears into your child's mind, but don't be surprised if he hasn't already worried about them himself. It is better to get these fears out in the open and offer suggestions for handling the unexpected than to wait until disaster strikes.

The previous example is not beyond the realm of possibility. In fact, it happened to young Jim.

In a tremendous hurry one morning, Jim's father dropped him off in the school parking lot. It never occurred to him that the school might not be open yet or that Jim would not know what to do if it weren't. When Jim's mother came home at noon that day, she found the first grader sitting on their doorstep. He had walked the two miles from the school and was waiting for her. He had not thought to wait at school. He had not thought to go to a neighbor's house. He didn't want to bother anybody. All he could think of to do was go home. He felt safe on the front steps. He was fine. But he needed to have been prepared for this unexpected event.

Over the course of weeks and months of daily discussions, your child will begin to feel safe enough to express fears that will afford opportunities for scriptwriting and rehearsals. You can also submit scenarios for discussion.

- What if you get lost in the mall? Which stores would you feel comfortable going into to ask for help? Which adults are okay to ask for help? What will you say?

- What if you come home on the bus and I'm not there because I had a flat tire? Which neighbor will you go to? What will you say? What if *she's* not there?

- What if your teacher asks you to sing a song in class? If you don't want to, how will you express that without feeling bad about yourself? If you want to sing, how will you do it?

- What if you go home with a classmate one afternoon, and you've never been to his house before? What will you say to his mother? What will you do while you are there? How can you ask where the bathroom is? What if you are hungry and no one offers you any food? What if your classmate ignores you? What if your classmate wants to play a game you don't want to play?

- What if the phone rings and I'm outside and don't hear it? Will you answer it? What will you say? What is scary about answering the phone? What's the worst thing that can happen?

- What if you get sick at school? How will you let your teacher know?

The goal is anticipating the unexpected is to give your child skills to cope in any situation. With enough practice in the safe environment of your daily discussions, he will gain confidence in his ability to handle anything, and he will become less anxious in general.

Weighing Desire and Risk

As you get to know your shy child, you can remind her of past problems in order to help her solve them. Suppose, for example, your fourth grader has been invited to a sleep-over with several other girls. The last time there was a sleep-over, you were called at 11:00 P.M. to come and get your daughter because she had been crying for a half hour and was in danger of becoming hysterical. You know that your child wants to go to this sleep-over, but you also know there is a good chance she won't make it, will embarrass herself, and will have further cause for negative self-talk in the future.

The daily discussion is a great place to bring up the topic of the sleep-over. If you haven't gone over the last sleep-over in a previous discussion, now is the time to do it. Review the scene. Encourage your child to talk about what happened and try to get her to remember at what point she began to think she could no longer stand to be there. What are her thoughts about what happened, and what negative self-talk is revealed by those thoughts? She might say:

- *I wanted to go to sleep and everybody kept talking.* (I never have anything to say. I thought they would laugh at me.)

- *Nobody was paying any attention to me.* (I thought they didn't like me.)

- *I was afraid I would wake up at night and not be able to find the bathroom.* (I'm afraid to ask questions. The others would be mad if I woke them up.)

- *I was afraid of her mother.* (I thought she would yell at me. I thought she didn't like me.)

- *I was hungry, but I didn't know how to ask for something to eat.* (I think people won't like me if I bother them.)

- *I had a stomachache.*

Once you have the problems and her thoughts about them on the table, you can begin to rewrite the scenario in ways that will lead to positive outcomes. You can change the scenario to the upcoming sleep-over and ask your child, for example, whom she would ask for something to eat and what words she would use. Do some "what-iffing." What if the mother says, "No, you can't have anything to eat"? What if the mother yells at you? What is the worst thing that could happen? How will you handle that? What if you start feeling sad again and want to come home? What can you do to avoid crying?

It is sometimes a good idea to steer the discussion in a direction that will help the child see that, in fact, she probably shouldn't go to the sleep-over. The temptation is to send the child out into the world, to encourage her to spread her wings. But by restraining her according to your best judgment, you might be allowing her to get a better handle on social skills before she attempts something so difficult as a sleep-over. Some parents have gone as far as to let the child know they will not come and pick her up late in the night, thus not enabling the behavior that ends in embarrassment and shame. In many cases, a child who knows she has no out will decide not to go.

On the other hand, after a brainstorming session where the worst- and best-case scenarios have been discussed, strategies for coping have been rehearsed, and negative self-talk has been pointed out and converted, your child might feel ready to sally forth with courage and determination. Although you have been careful to treat her concerns and fears with the utmost seriousness, she may realize that the worst-case scenarios are ridiculous. Abbie's mom would never yell at her if she asked for a banana. And there is a spare bed in Abbie's sister's room she could go and sleep in if she gets tired and the others don't want to go to sleep. Nothing will happen she cannot self-talk her way through, now that she knows how to change her self-talk from negative to positive.

SCRIPTWRITING, REWRITING, ROLE-PLAYING, AND REHEARSING

In the course of the daily discussions, you will come across events that your child found overwhelming for reasons he cannot identify. The immediate goal is to find solutions that can apply to similar, future situations. The ultimate goal is to help your child understand that, although he cannot always change or control what happens around him, he can change his own behavior in response to what is happening. To change, he must build his repertoire of communication skills.

When your child describes an uncomfortable situation, it's time to have some fun. Together you can rewrite the unpleasant scene, substituting a positive outcome for the negative one. You can create a script for the next time a similar situation arises. Then, if your child is willing, you can role-play or rehearse how the situation can be handled next time.

For example: Your child has told you that his second-grade class was paired with a sixth-grade class during gym. The second graders were paired off with sixth-grade buddies. Each pair was supposed to come up with a game together and then play it with the whole group. Your child admits that, while the pairs were being matched up, he had a sudden stomachache that made him start to cry, and the teacher let him sit out.

Little by little you get the picture that as he watched all the fun, he realized that his stomachache wasn't so bad and he really wanted to play. By now, though, he didn't know how to get off the bench and join in. He hoped someone would come and ask him to play, but no one did. He hoped the teacher would come over and ask how he was doing and ask him if he was ready to join the group, but she was too involved in the games to notice him.

Your first task while considering this problem is to keep your poker face on. You've heard similar stories before. Maybe many times before. You suspect there was no stomachache to begin with. And yet the last thing you can do is challenge your child on the stomachache issue—*the very last thing*. Assume there was a stomachache. Depending on how far your child has come in talking about shyness, you might suggest that the stomachache was actually *related to* the shyness. But never say aloud that you doubt the reality of the pain.

To avoid making your child feel ashamed of his inability to interject himself into this scenario, blame the whole thing on shyness. That darned shyness! We're going to beat it and here's how:

Rewrite the scene. Rewrite it several different ways. Ask your child to say what might have happened. His first response might be:

- I walk into the gym; I see the sixth graders; my stomach hurts and I think I can't play. But I go ahead and play anyway.

Sounds great! You don't want to admit it to your child, but you doubt it's going to happen that way. Having established early on that you are going to rewrite the scene with several different endings, you can move on from here. Establish that the imagination is king, and every possibility will be entertained. Have fun. Develop the worst- and best-case scenarios. These are some of the scenes he may imagine:

- I'm sitting on the bench. I feel better. I really want to play but I think it's too late. I get up and go to the teacher and say, "I'm feeling better now," or "I'm ready to play now." Let your child imagine all the possible things the teacher might say and how he could respond.

    —*Sorry, it's too late. You can't play now.* (What would you do if she said that? "Just go back and sit down, I guess.")

    —*Okay, John, go and ask that boy over there if he will be*

your partner. (What would you do? "I think my stomach would start hurting again." Yes, but what could you do? "I could ask the teacher to ask him." What if she gets mad?)

—*Okay, John, I'll ask Richard to be your partner.*

—*Okay, John, but all the sixth-grade boys are taken as partners. You can join James and Richard and there will be three of you!*

—She hugs you and tells you she's glad you are feeling better.

• I'm sitting on the bench. I'm feeling better. I decide I want to play. I don't see any sixth-grade boys who don't have partners. The teacher is busy and she hates to be interrupted. I go up to my best friend and his sixth-grade partner and ask if I can play with them.

—What's the worst thing that could happen. How would you handle it?

—What is likely to happen?

—What else *could* happen?

• The only person without a partner is a sixth-grade girl. He says, "Mom, I would never, never, never go up to a sixth-grade girl and ask her to play with me." You say, "Can't say I'd blame you."

In all likelihood, after a number of sessions like this one, your child will probably realize that the far-out answers are unlikely, that anyone he approaches will probably help him, but that even if they don't and he gets rejected, he has a contingency plan.

Throughout this process, keep your ears open for negative self-talk, and be prepared to point it out to your child later. You can say, "When we were talking about your approaching the teacher, I heard you say, 'The teacher will probably think I'm crazy (stupid, faking).' Does that sound like negative self-talk to you?" You might point out that the negative self-talk—the fear of what the teacher would think of him—is what kept him from getting up and entering the games. It is not wise to ask an impossible-to-answer question like, "Why do you assume she would think something bad of you?" It is much better to suggest ways your child can turn that negative thought around next time. ("The teacher likes me. The teacher will be glad to see me in the game. It's going to be okay.")

After you come up with various scripts that rewrite the scene, you can role-play the possibilities. Choose the easiest solution first in order to gain immediate success and build the confidence to move on to the next, more complex solution. For fun, include the worst-case scenarios. You can play the big, bad teacher or rude sixth-grade boy to the hilt.

PLANNING FOR FUTURE EVENTS

In the early elementary years, your child might not be able to express anxiety over upcoming events. It might even take a few years before you recognize the signals that let you know she is worrying about the future. If you can attach the behavior to the self-talk that is the constant companion of your shy child—if you can realize what a large part her imagination is playing in her preparation for special events—then you can help her during your daily discussions to anticipate how the situation will really play out, warn her about possible mishaps, and help her rehearse how she will handle those unexpected disasters.

Later in the elementary school years children gain the ability to imagine the worst-case scenario quite well on their own. If your child is open about her fears, it makes your job easier. When she lets you know something is coming up, spend some time "what-iffing" with her. Get silly. Get serious. Come up with solutions. Let her talk step by step about how she thinks the event is going to unfold. Have her imagine all the people she will have to interact with. What will they say? What will she say? Rehearse.

When anticipating a dress-up parade, a trip to the fire station, or any event that is out of the ordinary, some shy children begin imagining exactly how the event will happen. They build up the event in their minds. They plan their role, what they will wear, and sometimes all this planning is blown entirely out of proportion. Some children create a pretty scene surrounding an event which has them at center stage. Before a dress-up parade, for example, a shy child might fantasize about her costume being the best in the show. She might imagine how all the parents and teachers who see the parade will come to her and tell her how wonderful it is and how the other kids will admire her at last and see that she is wonderful. This kind of planning can produce anxiety, and it can also set the child up for disappointment. When the slightest thing goes wrong—a forgotten hat, a missing veil—or when she realizes that, in fact, there are so many costumes that she is not really going to stand out in the crowd at all, the stomachache begins, the tears fall, and refusal to participate in the parade is even possible.

Other shy children, faced with an unusual event, might suppress their anxiety about it altogether, so that when the event occurs they have no expectations. The danger is that they are frequently surprised by the amount of energy it takes to go through with the event. This too can lead to refusal, tears, and even panic.

To rehearse upcoming events, have your child describe the scenario as she thinks it will play out. Listen for any negative self-talk—any indication that she thinks she is inadequate for the play, the parade, the field trip. You can write anticipated problems down on index cards, and for each problem brainstorm solutions, writing those down on separate cards. Then you can ask her to pick a card, and the two of you can role-play the scenario with that solution.

You want your child to look realistically at the coming event and to plan for mishaps that might lead to a shy reaction that will embarrass her or make her miss out on some fun.

THE GOAL

All the examples of problems shy children face in elementary school have one thing in common. They are related to the child's unwillingness to make her needs known or to communicate effectively with others. Though shy children typically are very articulate, they usually lack good communication skills. The shy child's extreme sensitivity to any type of evaluation and her emerging emphasis on the differences between herself and others, which she might interpret as her not fitting in, lead her to avoid situations where there is any chance those differences might lead to a negative reaction from authority figures or peers. A shy person might have penned the famous admonition "Better to keep your mouth shut and be thought a fool, than to open it and have it known."

The major goal for these elementary years, then, is for the shy child to learn that the rewards of communicating with others outweigh the risks. Teaching this concept might not be easy because, in order to succeed, a child must be ready to acknowledge that his behavior is causing him discomfort. Usually it is you, the parent, who will be able to identify the source of that behavior as shyness, and you must be able to help the child understand it also. Though some children really don't want to communicate with others (some are genuinely unsocial), shy children do usually sense that there is some secret to human interaction that they do not know; some skill they are lacking. If you can help your child understand that communication is a skill that can be learned even in the face of extreme shyness, you will have started your child on the road to improved self-esteem and confidence.

Remember: It is best to not set a goal toward "curing" shyness. In Part I we emphasized that shyness is a personality style, not a personality disorder. But here we will see that the behaviors a shy child begins using during the elementary years to cope with shyness *can* be changed to make social interactions more comfortable. The process is often esteem-building. One mother of an elementary school child describes her daughter as becoming brave during the process of learning to communicate with others. "She will always be shy," says the mother. "But now I see her lift her chin and force her eyes to meet another's eyes. And she is proud of herself later because she knows she is courageous."

The journey toward understanding and managing shyness, when traveled together by you and your child, leads to a closeness usually not shared between outgoing, outward-looking children and their parents. To help your child you must know what has happened, what is happening, and what is going to happen in his daily school schedule. In the process of helping him, you learn about his interior life, and you learn to appreciate the delightful observations he makes on life viewed from his watchful place. Your child learns to let his rich imagination fly. He learns that it is safe to express what he is thinking; that his parents don't think he's weird; and that, probably, no one else does either. He learns to trust himself and his thoughts because you trust and value him. And you learn more about your child as an individual than most parents ever hope to know.

CHAPTER SUMMARY

1. Elementary school presents enormous challenges to the shy child.

2. Starting at age six, children develop an independent sense of self. Shy children often see themselves as separate from others.

3. Giving your child an advance tour of her school will help make the first days and weeks there much easier.

4. Your child will feel more comfortable if he can meet his teacher before school starts.

5. Getting to know your child's teacher will help the two of you work as allies as you support your shy child.

6. There are many new kinds of social situations outside of the classroom that your child must learn to cope with.

7. Asking friendly, open-ended questions during the daily discussion is the key to understanding what is going on in your child's life at school.

8. Role-playing can be enormous fun for both parent and child at this age.

9. The goal during these years is to help the shy child develop good communication skills.

Chapter 8

THE MIDDLE SCHOOL YEARS

If you are like most parents, it may seem to you that the transition your child makes from elementary school student to preteenager happens overnight. One day you have a child who begs you to play hopscotch with her; the next you have a quasi-stranger in your house who prefers time in her room alone. To confuse you further, a preteen can ricochet back and forth across the personality spectrum—acting like a happy child, a dissatisfied stranger, a pseudomature teen, then back to your little one—all in the course of one afternoon.

Parenting any middle-school-aged child can be exhausting. Outgoing children often have to be held back. Parents have to put the brakes on a child who wants to grow up too soon—to conform to the adult world too quickly. Shy children may have other needs. Remember the preschooler who couldn't express his feelings and whose frustration grew until it exploded in temper tantrums? The emotional roller coaster that is preadolescence confronts your child with much more powerful feelings, and he is likely to enter a new phase where it is harder than ever to sort out what he is feeling. More than ever before, your shy child needs you to learn how to communicate with him. And your learning to communicate will call for more than the usual amounts of patience and sensitivity.

All children need their parents to stay the course of pursuing common interests, make time to talk together every day, and maintain a healthy level of involvement. Adolescence is naturally a period when every child begins to feel increasingly self-aware, to become sensitive to the need for peer acceptance, and to recognize the need to achieve a degree of independence from parents. Could there be three more difficult emotional mountains for a shy child to climb? It is as if someone said, "Okay—let's take those parts of the shy child's personality that are the most difficult to moderate; then we'll design the teenage years so that the spotlight burns on those very issues!" Have you heard the words "You don't understand me! You don't understand what I'm feeling!" lately? Relax; you are in good company. Let's take a look at what is going on inside your shy child. When you have a more objective understanding of his feelings and what he's thinking, you will know how to respond in a loving, constructive way.

THE TOUGHEST YEARS

It can be hard for parents to differentiate between the normal changes of adolescence and those behavioral changes that result from a child's shyness. To make matters more confusing, a nonshy elementary child can start to show strong introverted characteristics during preadolescence. Some parents of middle school children may find themselves dealing with shyness issues for the first time, feeling all the more baffled because their child made it through elementary school seeming self-confident and outgoing.

Emotional Changes

The tough emotions that we normally associate with adolescence—feeling awkward, lonely, moody, estranged, and angry—take children by surprise when they begin to surface during the middle school years.

Conformity. One contributor to frustration and mood swings in middle schoolers is the powerful urge to conform to the group. Your shy middle school child may seem desperate sometimes in his need to avoid acting or looking different. He does not want to stand out in any way. Unfortunately, his strong observation skills make him painfully aware of differences, and his poor social appraisal skills may convince him that others are staring or laughing at him, when in fact they are doing nothing of the sort.

To minimize the potential for this kind of stress, it is worthwhile to spend extra money and buy your shy child a few outfits that are popular styles with her classmates, as long as they are in keeping with the values of your family. Like it or not, middle school children judge each other by the clothes they wear, and this evaluation is sharpest during the first weeks of school when most students rely on superficial assessments while trying to sort out the social scene. If you are not aware of what children consider appropriate clothing, it is a good idea to spend some time in the local mall or some other popular teen spot to get a sense of what the fashion style is. Until now you might have brought clothes home for your children and met with little resistance. It's time, though, to stand aside and let your child choose her own wardrobe. If all goes well, she will feel less out of place when school starts, and will fit in better, on the surface at least.

Nonconformity. Paradoxically, the desire to conform is often at odds with the young adolescent's equally powerful desire to establish himself as an individual with a unique identity. With keenly developed powers of observation, some shy children recognize fairly quickly that clothing and hairstyles are superficial ways to gain acceptance. They soon realize that there is much more to the game. If your shy child feels estranged from the predominant social groups at school—if he feels he cannot break into any group—don't be surprised if he appears to be taking the tack away from conformity. He may express disdain toward groups, sneering at the "lemmings" or the cliques who move through the halls in loud packs.

Perhaps you applaud this behavior and feel pleased that your child is not automatically going along with the crowd. Or perhaps it disturbs you that this behavior might further alienate him from social groups that are important to you. Either way, it will help you to realize that it is the rare child who genuinely wants to be a loner. In most children who respond to social stress by rejecting the whole notion of society, underneath the disdain is an aching need to belong to some group. It is possible for a shy child to combine the two seemingly opposing needs—the need to conform and the need to individuate—by joining up with a group that reflects his own *interests* as opposed to yours (see "Getting the Shy Middle Schooler Involved," p. 201).

Between Parent and Child. Your shy early adolescent is a bundle of exposed nerves. Most parents find it easy to become angry when it seems every other interaction is fraught with tension. Parents report feeling that they are walking on eggshells around their children, never knowing when an innocent remark will be taken the wrong way. Given patience and confidence on your part, however, there is a way to help your child get off the emotional roller coaster that is preadolescence. Psychologist Carl Rogers calls for an attitude of "unconditional positive regard." What he means is that you love your child when she is yelling at you, you love her when she is refusing to speak to you, and you make your parenting decisions based on what is in the best interest of the child and not when you are in a state of personal emotional reaction to her behavior. You continue to convey to your child, in spite of bizarre behavior, that you are on her team. In that way, you build trust.

Personality Changes

If you have been working with your shy child for a while, you already know that it is normal for him to withdraw on occasion in order to regroup. During early adolescence, you may be startled to see that when he reemerges from a period of social time-out, he has adopted a new personality. It is entirely normal for adolescents to try on new ways of being. As one mother of a twelve-year-old put it, "I never know when I wake up in the morning who I'm going to be having breakfast with."

Of course, a total withdrawal, the adoption of a violent or self-destructive personality, or any discussion of suicide require immediate attention and the help of professionals. But temporary attempts to take on a personality that keeps the world at bay are not at all unusual and usually are not permanent. They are just a normal part of adolescent experimentation. For shy children, personality changes are often attempts to place a veil of solitude around themselves.

The Human Burr. The Human Burr keeps others at a distance by acting like a complete pain in the neck. Rather than be hurt, the Burr becomes obnoxious, whiny, and irritable. The Burr may also use bad hygiene as a defense mechanism. He figures if he smells bad enough or doesn't wash his hair, maybe people will leave him alone. The Burr knows that interpersonal contact makes him uncomfortable, and he is willing to go to extreme lengths to limit such contact. He still wants a friend, and can be quite soft on the inside, but on the surface he is touchy and rude.

The Shy Rebel. This is the brooding loner, a James Dean kind of character. Sometimes this persona unintentionally becomes attractive to peers. Others may perceive the Rebel as mysterious or charismatic, particularly if he or she is good-looking. Your Shy Rebel may be terribly confused by this. He does not feel popular or believe that anyone would want to get to know him better. He does not feel connected or cool. If he has the strength to be independent or to rebel openly in a constructive way, then it should be relatively easy to help guide him into a few meaningful relationships or a rewarding after-school activity.

The Nerd. One mother of a shy preteen asked her daughter to describe the social makeup of her sixth-grade class. Her daughter had a perfect picture of what the groups were and where everyone fit in and why. When she asked where the daughter thought she herself fit in, the mother was shocked to hear her say, "Oh, I'm one of the weirdos." More shocking than the daughter's perception of herself as weird was the impression she gave that she was very pleased with the distinction.

The Nerd is a common personality for shy preteens to adopt. Preteen Nerds tend to be loners. They avert their eyes and talk to few of their peers. They put up with the tormenting behavior of others by trying to ignore it, and they rarely report the harassment. Because they are more comfortable talking to adults, Nerds can easily hold conversations with their teachers, which does little to improve their standing in the eyes of their fellow students. However, if there are other students in the class who are shy and perceive themselves as Nerds, then these students often form a bond that can become quite strong and healthy over time—as long as the children do not adapt dangerous behaviors in order to further set themselves apart.

The Blank Slate. Some shy children are so anxious about the impression they might leave on others that they project no personality at all. This shy middle schooler comes across as a blank slate with no definable characteristics. This is not a good strategy.

Several psychological studies have shown that if a person does not define himself for a group, the group will develop a negative impression of the person. Humans fear the unknown. We are suspicious of someone who averts her eyes, mumbles, or shies away from contact. Once the group has singled out a shy child to be picked on, others who may have been inclined to offer friendship are afraid to step forward, knowing that they may also become the butt of jokes and teasing.

Despite your shy child's natural inclination, she should

not keep a low profile. It may come as a shock to her, but you need to explain that her reticence makes other people anxious. Kids make fun of the unknown, in part, to deal with feelings of uneasiness. Middle schoolers, with their strong need for conformity, need to categorize people. Your shy child is hard to categorize because she does not offer up any information about herself. Your work with your shy middle schooler will help her define her own personality so that it opens her up to friendships, makes her proud and comfortable, and gives her an identity.

SHOULD WE MOVE?

For some shy children, middle school is more than tough; it is torture. Families with children who have withdrawn to the point that they absolutely refuse to communicate, refuse to go to school, or are being tormented by others, may be tempted to take the drastic step of moving their household to another school district in the hopes of giving their children a chance to start over.

Moving helps only if it is coupled by a strong commitment within the family to a) improve the parents' relationship with the child, and b) help the child work through his shyness issues at the child's pace, and with the child's active cooperation. Without such a commitment, after all the time, expense, and upheaval of a move, the pattern is likely to repeat itself in a new school. If you have gotten to the point where you feel that moving is your only solution, you may need to consider working with a professional to strengthen family relationships and help your child develop self-confidence and pride.

STARTING SCHOOL

Most school districts do a less than adequate job preparing elementary school students for middle school. Students may get a tour in the late spring and, if they are lucky, will have an orientation a day or two before school actually starts. Your shy child needs more.

As with all new places your shy child must get used to, preparation is the key to success. The more chances your child has to visit the middle school before he starts attending there, the less anxious he will be when school starts. As parent, you will need to be proactive in initiating these visits.

If your child has an older sibling at the school, then your job is made easier. Volunteer for activities that take place in the evening—work the snack stand during basketball games, sell cakes after orchestra concerts, help in the parking lot during homecoming—and be sure to have your soon-to-be-middle schooler tag along. As you know, shy children are hyperobservant. You want the building, the halls, the library, cafeteria, rest rooms, and gym to become familiar places.

At a minimum, drive past the middle school several times during the summer in a pressure-free situation. Do not say things like "There it is, James. Thirty-seven days and you'll be walking through those doors." He is well aware of it. Try to use the athletic fields or track during the summer. Contact the principal at the end of the summer and ask to bring your child before the school officially opens so he can meet the principal and as many staff members as possible. Just wandering the empty halls will help your child avoid embarrassment during the first few days of school when he must negotiate changing classes with hallways full of students.

Lunch

Lunch is one of the worst times of the day for shy adolescents. Once they get out of elementary school, they say goodbye to cafeterias with assigned seating and adult supervision. Lunchtime is an intensely social time. The shyest preadolescents will sometimes take drastic measures to avoid having to find a place to sit in the cafeteria or the humiliation of sitting alone. They will go to the school nurse or hide in the bathroom, hang around the school office or find an empty classroom to sit in. It will not take teachers long to figure out what is going on. If you get wind of such behavior on your child's part, though there are no easy solutions you can help her plan what she is going to do during lunch period.

If you are not shy and have never felt the devastating loneliness of being in a large room with a hundred people, not one of whom you feel you can approach, then you will need to develop an attitude of patience and compassion. It is easy enough to say to your child, "Just walk up to some members of your class and sit down. That's what they expect you to do." But for your shy child, such a seemingly simple act is beyond the realm of possibility.

As with previous shy behaviors, one of the best things you can do for your child is to model social skills. If you can, attend covered-dish suppers or other food-related events with your child, and speak with her beforehand about what you are going to do to make a place for yourselves at a table. Then do it. You can also go over the specific words she can use as she joins a table of classmates and give her specific language for conversation starters. Though it is important to remain positive and upbeat when imagining scripts of this kind, it is also necessary to be realistic about the behavior of some middle schoolers. Your child might generate the courage to approach a table of her peers, and one or more of those peers might rebuff her. They might even be cruel about it. In your daily discussions (see p. 209) be prepared to process episodes where your child is rejected and to offer her suggestions for how to respond.

You can also suggest to her that if she does sit alone, her body language can either encourage or discourage others from joining her. That is, if she keeps her eyes down on the table while she eats, if she puts her books and papers all over the table, or if she reads a book during lunch, she will not invite companionship. If, on the other hand, she leaves the table free of clutter and the chairs pulled out and looks around the room with interest while she eats, eventually someone is likely to join her, perhaps another shy person for whom finding a place to sit is equally difficult.

It is wise to discuss the lunchroom with your child before middle school starts. Otherwise the sensation of entering the cafeteria with no guidelines about where to sit may come as a genuine shock to her. When school starts, have her take a packed lunch for at least the first week. That reduces the stress of the unfamiliar lunch line, and allows her to control what she eats. As she develops friendships in extracurricular activities, help her rehearse how to ask someone to eat lunch with her before they get into the lunchroom.

GETTING THE SHY MIDDLE SCHOOLER INVOLVED

The key to middle school success for the shy child is *involvement*. You must insist, in a loving way, that your child involve herself in some kind of ongoing school activity, such as band, the school newspaper, a sports team, or an outside extracurricular activity such as dance, volunteering, or a religious group. Ideally, some of the children in her extracurricular activity will be her classmates at school. You need to make your feelings about outside activities clear as early as possible, with language like, "When you start middle school, which activity do you think you'll sign up for?" The assumption is that she *will* be signing up for something. It is a quiet, constant assumption, just as you assume your child will brush her teeth and do her homework.

If your shy preteen panics at the thought of joining a group, then you can point out that everyone needs balance in life. Just as it is not healthy for an adult to devote every waking minute to one job with no hobbies or outside interests, it is not healthy for a middle school student to take care of the academic work in her life without some kind of outside activity. As always, you can model good behavior here. Kids this age are extremely sensitive to hypocrisy. Make sure that you make time for some type of activity that you love—the gym, group outings to the museum, golf—before you lay the law down to your child. Watching television or playing on the computer does not count as a legitimate extracurricular activity for you or your child.

The best activity for your child is one that stems naturally from his own interests. Get a copy of the activities available from the middle school office early in the summer and go over it with your child. If nothing is appealing, then explore your community with your child in search of something that attracts him. You may run into resistance that needs to be worked through with brainstorming and rehearsing scenarios. Above all, maintain your calm insistence that this is something your child will do. Your child does not get to choose whether or not he is involved in an extracurricular activity; he does, however, get to choose the activity.

How to Start

Before you can involve your shy middle schooler in an activity, you have to have a meaningful relationship with him. If you don't, then your pronouncement "You will join X" might be greeted by stubborn refusal, and no one wins that war. Assuming you have been working on the relationship with your child, enjoying activities together, working side by side at family chores, and learning about each other's interior lives, then you can put your foot down and insist.

Even if you have a close relationship with your shy child, you may run into some resistance. Be patient and firm. Offer to accompany your child. Brainstorm with your child about a buddy or acquaintance that he could ask to join him. Rehearse what it might feel like to walk into the newspaper club meeting, the lacrosse practice, or the dance studio for the first time. Remember to keep things playful as you imagine all the ridiculous disasters that could happen, as well as the more mundane truth. Let your child talk about what might run through his mind, and point out his negative self-talk. Try to help him to acknowledge it if his self-talk is talking him out of joining.

Band. Of all the activities available to shy preteens, joining the band is one of the best things they can do. Band allows children to express themselves through music. The children in the band are usually a tightly knit group. The band tends to be a healthy and safe social atmosphere; it can be a godsend for shy children. Band is highly structured; it allows shy children to be in the presence of their peers, but to relate to them musically—and the notes they are supposed to play are right in front of them. Band provides a handy topic of conversation if your child can't think of anything to say. Playing an instrument and sitting behind a music stand often give the shy adolescent comfortable buffers that allow him to relax a bit in the company of others. Even if your middle school child has never played an instrument, if he shows an interest, it is worth it to sign him up for lessons in the summer so he can join in the fall. Playing in the band may change his life.

Art. Early adolescents with artistic talents can easily shape their identity around those skills. Make sure that your shy middle schooler is introduced to the art teacher by taking him for a quiet meeting with the teacher before or after school at the beginning of the year. The art room can become a home away from home for the shy child. Many schools offer artistic children the chance to paint scenery for plays, to decorate lobbies, and to display their art in the halls. Shy artists can often better communicate through their art than with the spoken word. Most importantly, your shy artists will find companionship in the company of other artists in the art room.

If your middle schooler doesn't like drawing, try putting a camera in her hands. Taking pictures for the yearbook or school newspaper is an ideal activity for shy children. It is an individual activity that has a few group meetings. The camera provides a legitimate buffer for the photographer, giving her permission to look at other people and involve herself in a safe, modulated way. The camera gives her something to do with her hands and provides structure. Best of all, most peo ple like to have their pictures taken, and photographers often become popular and appreciated.

Make sure your shy preteen stays organized if she's involved in a deadline activity. She may put off an assignment or two if she is anxious about the social contact required. If she doesn't do her job, and the newspaper or yearbook is delayed because of it, she'll face negative social consequences that could discourage her from ever joining a group activity again.

Sports. Erin was so shy she put up with girls stealing her hair bands right off her head for months before telling anyone. She was too embarrassed to use the bathroom at school. And she hated it when other people looked at her—hated it so much she was uncomfortable eating in restaurants.

Erin was tall, as were both of her parents. They enrolled her in the recreational basketball league and installed a basketball hoop in their driveway. Before each practice and game, they gave Erin only one thing to think about. One week it was "Keep your arms up," the next it was "Rebound." Her height compensated for her relative lack of skill and discomfort on the court.

Despite her anxiety about performing, Erin kept playing. She drilled alone in the driveway and studied women's basketball games on television. Her parents could tell her confidence was growing when she stopped hugging herself during time-outs and stood up straight with her hands on her hips. Erin began to have small successes; she learned how to rebound, she loved the roar of approval when she blocked a shot, and she developed enough confidence to try to make a basket when she got the ball.

As her athletic skill improved, her parents offered social

tips. Erin learned how to congratulate teammates on a good play, how to look at her coach's face and nod when she was talking, and how to talk casually after practice. It took a few years, but the confidence that started to grow in the gym carried over to Erin's life at school. She had an identity: She played basketball, and she was becoming a very good player. She belonged to a group, and children looked up to her (in more ways than one). She was still a reserved girl, introspective and somewhat quiet. But the day Erin joined a new summer league team and *she* was the one who took charge of introductions and directing the warm-up (with no adult intervention), her mother almost burst into tears. Through sports, her daughter was learning to express and assert herself.

Many shy middle schoolers reject the idea of joining a sports team outright; sports are unpredictable, your teammates have great expectations of you (increasing your chances of failure), you have to perform in front of large groups, and the physical stimulation and noise can be overwhelming. Sports also conjure up bad memories of horrendous gym class experiences.

Do not dismiss sports, however. As you enjoy your daily discussions with your shy adolescent, explore what his sports fantasies are. Does he ever dream of being a World Series pitcher? An Olympic fencer? A polo player, rugby star, gymnastics stand-out? If he enjoys exercise, he may prefer a sport that allows him to perform as an individual for the team's benefit, such as golf, swimming, or track.

Sports build physical confidence, which in turn can affect the way a middle schooler sees himself. He doesn't have to transform himself overnight into the star quarterback. But he may enjoy the challenge of learning something new, as well as the pleasant physical sensations and rewards of exercise. If your child has not participated in sports before, be cautious about having him join a team where the other kids have been playing for years. His relative lack of skills and knowledge of the game will compound his social anxiety. Further, his expectations will not be met, and he will be likely to drop out. Can he lift weights at the local gym? Learn racquetball? How about bicycling or skiing? Be creative. Research the opportunities in your community as well as the middle school.

Dance. Haley was terrified of talking to boys. As a way of distancing herself from people, she stubbornly insisted on dressing in hippie clothes while everyone else in her school dressed in preppy fashions. Shy in elementary schools, she entered into a deep depression when middle school began and isolated herself from her family. She was the girl the others picked on and teased. She had no self-esteem, and no sense of direction.

Haley's parents were surprised when she chose dance as her extracurricular activity. Haley was insistent; not just any kind of dance, it had to be classical ballet. It took a few tries to find a dance studio where Haley felt comfortable and an instructor who seemed the right fit, but Haley didn't give up. The studio quickly became Haley's home away from home and she begged for more lessons. Her depression reduced dramatically. As she danced, she lost weight and developed a strong, striking figure. She did not develop a close friendship with any girls at her school, but she had many friends at the dance studio. The positive social experiences at the studio became an anchor and softened the difficulties of school. By age fourteen, she had a circle of kind, supportive friends and had started seeing a nice boy who valued her dance, her quirky clothes, and everything about her.

Younger dancers looked up to her. Haley had found her niche; she made a place for herself with the support of her family.

Dance appeals to shy middle schoolers because of the degree of independence and autonomy it offers. They can choose between individual and group instruction. They develop body confidence in front of the mirror before they have to perform in front of others. If you find the right instructor, there is no performance pressure, but the chance to grow and learn is paced to the child's ability and needs. As middle schoolers get into better physical shape, they are picked on less often, both because they carry their body with more confidence, and because they don't tolerate harassment.

Developing Other Skills Outside of School. If your child is handy, let him work on your car. In a few years, being able to do simple engine repair will make him a very popular person. Arrange for your child (with his permission, of course) to tutor a younger child in an academic area he excels in. He will gain a tremendous boost by helping the child and will be able to practice social skills on a less critical audience than his peers. Likewise, a sensitive child might want to volunteer at a retirement community. The library is a haven for some shy children and is another place with volunteer opportunities. If your child chooses the library, try to ensure that he will have interpersonal contact and will not be relegated to restacking books. A successful extracurricular activity will come out of your child's interests and desires. Listen carefully and help him choose something that is a good fit.

Community- Vs. School-Based Activities. The disadvantage of dance, volunteering in the community library, or other community-based activities for a shy child is that they have little impact on life at school. If your child joins the school band and makes her niche in the trumpet section, then she has a recognizable social place, and people who will sit with her at lunch. Even if she wins the Volunteer of the Year award from your local Chamber of Commerce, it will have no impact on her social status at school. If your child is willing to join a community activity, but resists joining one at school, then respect that. Remember: The only lasting growth you can expect from your child will take place at his own pace. Encourage his participation in the community-based activity. Try again to get him to join a school activity the following year.

THE DAILY DISCUSSION FOR MIDDLE SCHOOL

If you have already built a strong relationship with your shy middle school student, then the two of you will be able to talk through new situations as they crop up, and you can help him anticipate potential problems and prepare for them. If you feel that your middle schooler is keeping you out of his life, then you must work to reenter it. The most important thing you can do is to listen to your child. Listen without comment. Avoid the temptation to straighten out all his problems. Most important, listen without judging.

When you are actively listening to your child, you may want to make sure you understand what he's saying. Stop him occasionally and say something along the lines of, "I don't want to put words in your mouth, but it sounds like you are saying . . .". He may not want you to solve his problems or point out everything he did wrong, but if you can show that you are listening and respecting him, that will be meaningful.

The daily discussion is not the time to quiz about schoolwork or be nosy about budding friendships. Let your child's interests be your compass. If she likes a particular rock group, then listen to their music so you an discuss it intelligently. If your child likes rockets, then it's time for you to learn more about rockets. There is a wonderful feeling for both parent and child when a parent is secure enough to let the child teach her something she didn't know before.

It might be helpful to jot down a list of topics if *you* feel tongue-tied. Middle school children are prone to see the world in black-and-white terms, and they can develop passionate, sometimes ideal visions of how the world should be. What does he think about the latest political scandal? About homelessness? How would he change things if he were school principal, or governor? Don't squash your child's idealism by pointing out everything that is wrong with his argument; listen to him. As he talks to you, he is developing conversational skills and learning how to assert himself in a positive way.

A great time for your daily discussion is when you and your child are working at something side by side, such as cleaning the kitchen together or weeding the garden. Make sure that your shy child sits next to you in the car when you are driving somewhere and let him pick the radio station. Some parents make a habit of taking an early morning walk or bike ride with their child so they can start the day with a shared activity. Others find that watching a baseball game to-gether provides them with an easy time to talk. If your week-days are too rushed and unpredictable, then one solution is to schedule your child for a one-on-one breakfast every week-end.

Scriptwriting, Rewriting, Role-Playing, and Rehearsing

If you have established a routine for going over your child's shy responses with him, then he might be happy to continue these activities into middle school. It will be useful—if you have a shy middle schooler and have just picked up this book—to look at how the daily discussions and role-playing can be used for elementary school children.

Whether you are continuing the techniques or just getting started, realize that while the goals are the same as they were for an elementary-school-aged child, and the fundamental at-titude of "I'm on your team" is still extremely important, these strategies must be handled differently with a shy middle school student. Most twelve-year-olds will balk if you suggest a high structured role-play or rehearsal of the sort that works like a charm for an eight-year-old. The daily discussion with your preadolescent requires a little more finesse. Shy children are great saboteurs. If he senses that you are trying to get him to rehearse telling the cafeteria lady he'd rather have peaches instead of green beans, chances are he'll close his mouth and either leave the room or lose himself in a book, the computer, or the television.

The role-playing and scriptwriting of this age comes from your casual conversations with your child. Sit down while your child is watching MTV and ask who the guitar player is. If your child responds with any degree of enthusiasm, ask a few open-ended questions, or make leading remarks. "I wonder what it feels like to stand in front of forty thousand screaming fans. I wonder what he's thinking." When watching a movie with your child's favorite star, you could start a playful conversation with, "If he came over to dinner, should we serve meat loaf or macaroni and cheese?"

Do not make direct comparisons to your child's life. It can be extremely hard to resist this temptation. For example: Your shy child gives you a perfect description of how a television character should react in a typical shy situation—"He shouldn't just walk away from that guy; he should ask him for help. It's not like the guy is going to bite him or anything." You can't hold back, and you say, "If you can see how the guy on the show should act, why can't you do that yourself?" You must be more subtle with middle schoolers and let them come to their own conclusions at their own pace.

Shy children have wonderful imaginations and excel at fantasizing. If your child shares some of her fantasies with you, listen actively. You want to encourage your child to open up. You can learn a great deal about what's going on in your child's mind by listening to her fantasies, much as you learned about your five-year-old child by asking him to talk about his drawings. Fantasies about turning the tables on a bully, impressing someone she has a crush on, or singing the National Anthem to a standing ovation will give you a framework regarding what issues she is concerned with and how severe things are.

Shy children have too much practice imagining the worst possible thing that could happen. You can help them train their imaginations to create rewarding scenarios. It is exactly the same process as turning negative self-talk into positive self-talk. As your shy middle schooler shares fantasy scenarios with you, you want to act as a funnel, asking questions of your child so that he decides what is realistic and what he can actually say or do.

Samuel was constantly picked on by the jocks in his grade. He told his father of a revenge fantasy that involved stealing the jocks' clothes when they were in the shower and forcing them to run around naked. His father asked, "What else could you do to get back at these guys?" Samuel suggested putting Ben-Gay in their jockstraps or urinating in the whirlpool. His father asked what would happen if he did that, and Samuel replied he would probably get beat up again. The conversation continued with Samuel venting his frustrations and his father listening closely. His father finally asked what the jocks wanted of Samuel. "They don't want me to be such a wimp or to get out of gym class," his son answered. "What do you want?" his father asked. "I want to stop looking stupid in gym. I don't know how to play any of the games and they laugh at me."

Samuel's father allowed his son to be angry and vengeful, and to think up nasty alternatives; then he helped Samuel funnel his thoughts to a realistic level and then really hit on the issue—his son felt awkward in gym and other boys teased and hurt him because of it. The next step was to find a place for Samuel to improve his sports skills, through Saturday classes offered by the community college. Samuel's father also realized that he had never taken the time to teach his son how to throw and catch a baseball the way his father had done for him. When he saw how unhappy Samuel was, he stopped working on Saturdays and devoted that day to showing his son the fun side of sports.

BULLIES

Shy children are often the targets of bullies. The situation does not change when your child moves from elementary to middle school. If anything, it might get worse. Bullying is always a serious issue; some view it as even more serious in middle school because of the size of the bullies and the amount of danger they can inflict.

Bullying is harassment and should not ever be tolerated. Bullies can cause permanent psychological damage, making a shy child doubt himself even more, and making him appear as a pariah to his peers. Never treat bullying as "boys being boys" or "girls being catty." If your child is being bullied, you need to find out who is doing it and when it is taking place; then you need to work with your child and perhaps school authorities, to put a stop to it.

Shy preteens are often reluctant to admit they are being bullied because they see it as an admission of weakness. If you suspect something is wrong, talk to teachers or other parents. A good guidance counselor can be a terrific ally. If you share your suspicion that bullying is going on, a guidance counselor is in the position to do some detective work. The best defense against bullies is to help your shy child develop enough self-confidence to put a stop to the harassment himself. When you know that bullying is going on, be sure to bring up the topic in conversation and help your child brainstorm methods of dealing with it.

INTERNAL WORK

Helping your shy middle schooler gain a sense of self-confidence does not end in a climax at the end of eighth grade with your child standing on a stage thanking you for your patience and understanding. Growth comes in fits and starts. You won't see much of it because it happens internally.

It can be frustrating to watch your shy early adolescent go through the same painful scenario time and time again. By this age they have language skill, they have some degree of logic, and you may feel all they are lacking is willpower. Many parents impose themselves on their child at this point, insisting that they act a certain way or forcing them into social situations that become nightmarish.

Your child must come to basic realizations about shyness and her ability to manage it on her own. The goal is to give your child plenty of chances for the great "A-ha!"—the moment of enlightenment when she realizes that another girl *will* respond favorably to an invitation to sit together at lunch, or that the world will not stop spinning if she smiles at someone. The power of the "A-ha!" cannot be overemphasized. You cannot say it for your middle school child. She won't tolerate it, or even believe it. But when she sees for herself what works and what doesn't, and when she sees it in the context of self-confidence in her ability to operate out of a shy personality, then she can begin to enjoy the social aspects of middle school.

Success in managing shyness requires flexible parents who see the process of parenting a shy child as an opportunity for self-growth. As your child matures and learns more about himself, you learn more about yourself through your involvement with the process and your ability to set up a few props and then step back and watch how your child handles them. Remember that your goal is not to change your child—not to transform a shy child into a nonshy one. In fact, you court disaster if you keep that goal going into adolescence. Your priorities are best placed in helping your child realize his highest potential within the framework of his basic personality style.

CHAPTER SUMMARY

1. Middle school (early adolescence) is the hardest age for all children and can be excruciating for shy children.

2. The shy child's normal hypersensitivity is even stronger during the middle school years.

3. Helping your shy child become comfortable with the middle school building will go a long way toward making the transition to middle school easier.

4. Shy children may develop several personality types to distance themselves from others.

5. Shy middle schoolers present a blank slate which leads other students to incorrect, negative assumptions.

6. Involvement in extracurricular activities is the key to social comfort in middle school.

7. Daily discussions with your shy middle schooler should be regular and relaxed.

8. Middle schoolers resist highly regimented rehearsal and

scriptwriting sessions. Parents must use a conversational approach to be successful.

9. Shy middle school children can only grow at their own pace, and much of the growth is internal.

Chapter 9

THE HIGH SCHOOL STUDENT

High school is the time for you to gently steer your shy teen, not to command or pressure him, even though shyness issues can acquire a level of urgency now. If your middle schooler was too nervous to talk to members of the opposite gender, now you're worried he'll graduate from high school without having gone on a date. Your timid twelve-year-old never gave you any worries by staying out too late, but now you realize that she has no friends. It becomes harder to intervene in your shy child's life because most adolescents, by definition, distance themselves from their parents. The clock is ticking; you only have a few years left to help before your shy child moves away and must face the world.

THE GOOD NEWS ABOUT TEENAGERS

Now that your child is fourteen years or older, she can use her expressive capabilities and improved communication skills to talk to you directly about her social anxieties. You no longer must rely on your child's drawings, or interpret her self-talk from statements she makes while playing with puppets. Though some parents complain that their teenagers are uncommunicative, adolescents can, in fact, be extremely skilled at talking. As a parent, you must take the lead to ensure that you are the person your teenager wants to talk to.

The teenage years can be a time of tremendous richness and delightful growth for both parent and child. Sharing the world with your teenager, seeing it from his perspective, watching as he learns to conquer fears and achieve goals is the reward for your years of concern and hard parenting work. The idealism of youth can provide an antidote for adult cynicism. The energy of adolescents is breathtaking. You have a new companion, a new way to see the world.

The common cultural assumptions about teenagers seem to be focused on their rebellion, rage, and sloppy personal habits. Do not let this attitude color the way you see your own child. Adolescence is a time of growth and separation from parents, but that doesn't necessarily mean constant conflict and anger. Teenagers can have a wonderful sense of humor; they are energetic, loving, and kind. They move out of your life all too soon, so it makes sense to try to enjoy the time you have left with them.

THE BAD NEWS ABOUT TEENAGERS

The bad news? The techniques that have worked with your shy child up until now will not work as well now that he is an adolescent. That's because the days of your child viewing you as the fount of wisdom are over. Older adolescents, especially, begin to make adult judgments about their parents. They see us, for the first time, as human beings with faults, who are capable of mistakes. When it comes to shyness issues, they start to doubt our best-intentioned advice. They resist our attempts to help just as the social pressure on them intensifies and they prepare to leave the cocoon of the home for the wider world of college and work.

The developmental work adolescents must undertake is to become independent of parents while blending in with a peer group. When the inborn impetus to establish a peer group collides with their natural social awkwardness, shy teens can experience high levels of anxiety, and that can find expression in unhealthy behaviors. If you do not help your shy teen learn to manage his anxiety, he can turn into an unhappy young adult.

As with all developmental stages, understanding what is going on in your child's interior life makes it easier to tolerate her prickly side and to bring out her better qualities. You may find it difficult to accept that she is turning her primary focus away from you, but remember that if she does not pass through this developmental stage, it will come back to haunt her someday. If you work with your shy teen to control her anxious responses, it will be easier for her to manage the shift from a family-centered to a peer-centered person, and eventually to incorporate both family and friends into a full, rewarding life.

SCHOOL ISSUES

A common mistake parents of high school students make is to resist communicating with the school staff, usually because they are trying to give their children more responsibility and independence, or because they have become caught up in work that is less child-centered now that their children are older. This parental shift away from school involvement is problematic for shy children, and you should be prepared to be as communicative with the school personnel as is possible.

Get to know your child's teachers and guidance counselors. Be aware of what your child's schedule is, and what kind of homework is being assigned. During your shy child's freshman and sophomore years, have your child jot down the due dates of projects and presentations on the family calendar so you can help her plan and prepare for something that she might otherwise avoid thinking about. Later, you can let her take responsibility for her own schedule, but make sure she knows that you will be checking it from time to time. She must learn how to plan and prepare on her own before she leaves home.

Why is supervision necessary for children this age? If your shy child has entered a large high school with twenty-five or thirty children in a classroom, she is likely to have difficulty asking the teachers for clarification on assignments. Without your involvement, she may consistently misunderstand what she is meant to do, or she may become overwhelmed and not be able to sort out the work at the end of the day. If she receives poor marks because she was too shy to ask for help, she can enter a downward spiral regarding schoolwork.

When you go over assignments with her, you give her an opportunity to say whether or not the teachers' expectations are clear. If she is confused, you can help her, either by giving her the language and support she needs to ask for help, by suggesting she call a friend and talk over the assignment, or simply by using your own judgment. If the problem persists, you may need to intervene with the teacher, and the sooner you do so in the course of a semester the better.

Interest Groups

Just as in middle school, participation in extracurricular activities is a lifeline for a shy teen. There is no substitute for the healthy sense of belonging that comes from being part of an organized group or club.

The band or marching band is one of the best groups imaginable. If your teen doesn't have a musical background, there may still be a place for him helping the band care for equipment or carrying banners. In the marching band, your shy child has a highly structured role: Play this song, march to this place, then to that place. The experience of playing music relaxes and makes many teens open to socialization. Many marching bands take trips for competitions, participate in shows, and offer summer band camps. Perhaps best of all, the marching band gives the shy teen a positive identity, a social niche, and a place of comfort.

Paradoxically, it seems, many shy teenagers opt for dramatics as an outlet. There is something about taking on a character and performing a set piece in front of an audience that allows a shy person to escape the bounds of social anxiety. However, it is often difficult for a shy teenager to assert himself and take the step of auditioning. Your encouragement can help here. Or, if the problem seems insurmountable, your child can join the stage crew and help with lighting, sound, or prop design and management.

Allow your teenager to choose his activity based on his interests, but insist that he choose something. He can work for the yearbook, paste up the newspaper, play chess, or join a language club. Many schools offer clubs that allow students to explore career options. It doesn't matter what your shy child chooses, as long as it is an organized activity that will put him in contact with others and help to define him positively in the eyes of his peers.

Adolescence is a period of physical as well as developmental growth, and a child who has never shown an interest in sports before may secretly want to try out for a team. Shy children tend to be overanalyzers. Sports take them out of their heads and ground them in the physical world, forcing them to spend time away from the "I wish" fantasies that can eat up their days.

Many shy teens enjoy rewarding experiences on teams that focus on individual achievements, such as track, cross-country running, tennis, swimming, gymnastics, bowling, or golf. When they become more confident, they may try out for sports that require a team effort, such as basketball or field hockey. Some churches sponsor intramural sports leagues that are less competitive and more participation-centered than high school sports. The children in church leagues tend to develop a strong sense of camaraderie and to worry less about their performance.

Shy teenagers benefit from a solid grounding in their ethnic heritage. Participation in religious schooling, such as Greek or Hebrew schools, joining ethnically based social clubs, or helping prepare for festivals or parades is an excellent way for a child to interact with others.

Whatever your shy teen chooses, your job is to make it as easy as possible for her to remain committed. While remaining sensitive to the level of involvement she *wants* from you, your being willing to drive, to help out with costumes, or to otherwise volunteer your time might make the difference between her continuing with the activity long enough to become comfortable with the group, and her giving up within a few months.

When you child is using negative self-talk to talk herself out of going to a meeting—"I don't have anything to offer." "Nobody spoke to me last week." "I'd rather just watch TV"—the fact that you are driving a group or that you are expected to show up too can provide the impetus she needs to get there. Likewise your own negative responses to the time it takes for you to be involved—or the money—will give her an easy excuse for quitting. Be prepared to take an active role and an active interest in whatever extracurricular activity your child chooses.

Planning for College

Some shy teenagers cannot wait to go away to college. They feel trapped by their reputation in their high school and community. When they get to college, they reason, they start with a clean slate. They can exhibit whatever personality they want. It is often true that a teenager, one who is locked into a shy role throughout grade school and high school, blossoms overnight when he gets to college.

Others, however, may feel extremely anxious at the thought of going away to school. If parents are unresponsive to an anxious child's concerns, he may sabotage his grades or standardized test scores to ensure that he cannot get into whatever far-flung university his parents have their hearts set on.

Whatever your shy teen's feelings about college, you must let him, within your financial constraints, set the course. He will not have a successful college experience, academically or socially, if you do not allow him to make the decision about where to go to school.

Shy people are exquisitely sensitive to place, so you will

want to visit the colleges that he is considering even if they are local. Visiting during the summer will not give a good feeling of how the campus looks and sounds when it is teeming with students. Visit in the middle of the semester. Make sure your tour includes time in dorm rooms, library, and gym and a meal in the cafeteria.

If your child chooses a local college, encourage her to live on campus. It will add to your expenses, but it greatly increases the chances she will develop friendships and a wide social network of acquaintances that will make her college years more enriching and help set her up for a successful adult life. When it comes to a choice of dormitory arrangements, the more the merrier. If she has the chance, encourage her to sign up for a room that will have four, five, or six roommates. In a larger group, a quiet person can more easily find her place. She will be swept into group activities. If she has a single roommate and the two of them don't get along, it may be difficult for her to hook up with another person.

Some shy young adults choose to live at home while attending college. Many urban or community colleges work hard to establish social opportunities for commuters. You may have to help your child identify these opportunities for social development, and support your child in her decisions.

THE VALUE OF SUMMER CAMP

If you suspect that the thought of college, with dorm life and strangers as roommates, is too intimidating for your shy teen, then consider summer camp. College can be an overwhelming concept, but a week at a sleep-away camp is manageable. Shy children can start worrying about going away to college as early as sixth or seventh grade. If your shy teen has a positive experience of a sleep-away camp under his belt, the thought of moving in with strangers will be easier.

Your choice of camp should be based on your child's interests. Many summer camps are actually held on college campuses, with the campers staying in dorms and eating at the cafeteria. This is ideal.

Summer camp itself might seem intimidating to your child. It will be easier if you can find a friend who wants to go to the same camp. Most shy children do well at sleep-away camp if they are motivated and prepared for it. You may be surprised at how much your child can mature and grow in self-confidence in seven short days!

SOCIAL SKILLS TRAINING

If you have been working with your shy high school student for a while, she may be starting to develop friendships, or may find herself the member of a group of friends. If your child has never really had friends before, she may need to learn some social skills. These are the kinds of things that many outgoing children pick up intuitively. Shy kids are hampered by their poor social appraisal skills and may not learn some of the basics about how to act in a group without a bit of training.

If your shy adolescent shares frustration or anxiety about how to behave in a group, here are the four important points to go over with him:

- Enter a conversation quietly. When you sit down at the lunch table and your group of friends are already talking, just say "hello." Don't blurt out something that may be off-topic or distracting to the others.

- Listen and get a feel for the conversation. Who is doing most of the talking? What is the focus of discussion? Think about what you could add or ask about.

- Ask about other people in the group. People love to talk about themselves, and shy teenagers should take advantage of this.

- Do not play one-upmanship. This is particularly a danger for boys. Trying to establish a place for yourself by appearing better than the others will only earn you an isolated seat at lunch.

The danger of the approach to conversation described above is that the tentative child may stay silent the entire time and never contribute to the conversation of the group. This usually happens when the shy child is unsure when to break in to talk. But, as many people have learned, it is not always necessary to be talkative in order to be considered part of a group. Woody Allen said once that "Ninety percent of life is just showing up." There is a place in every circle of friends for a member who is introspective and quiet, just as there is a place for a talkative teen and a joker. Your teenager cannot and should not try to change her personality because of a perception that she has to be a certain way in order to fit in. She can and should expect that good friends will accept her for who she is. But she should be encouraged to speak up when she has something to say in order to avoid becoming something of a blank slate (see Chapter 8).

DATING

It is sometimes hard to tell who is more anxious about a shy teen's chances of getting a date—the teenager or his parents. Parents who had a less-than-perfect high school experience often try to live vicariously through their children. They want their shy child to be popular, appear normal, be involved, and date. They want their child to have what they didn't have.

This attitude is poisonous for a shy adolescent, only adding to his anxiety on this most sensitive of subjects. A number of shy teens go through high school without ever having been on a date. If this is true of your child, be aware that it may trouble him, and it may not. If he wants to ask someone out badly enough, it will probably become obvious to you and you might be able to help him work through the necessary steps. If the subject does not come up, however, it may be that he knows he is not ready and he has accepted it. As long as your shy teen is learning how to function comfortably in social situations, and he has a few friends, do not be alarmed if he doesn't go to the prom. Many shy teens blossom in college, and quickly catch up to their peers in terms of interactions with the opposite gender.

Like it or not, it is still true that the situation for girls and boys is different when it comes to dating. While more girls feel comfortable asking boys out, in the majority of cases the boy is still expected to take the initiative. This leaves a shy girl waiting. Where shy may become anxious is in figuring out how to let a boy know she is interested in him. Or she may be asked out and not know how to respond. Again, if you have reasonably good communication with your child, you will probably know when anxiety over this issue reaches a critical point.

If your shy adolescent does want to ask someone for a date, wants to learn to assert herself, or is asked out and isn't sure what to do, there are a number of things you can do to help.

Survey the Field. Many of the basic rules of dating are foreign concepts to adolescents, particularly those who do not have wide or strong social contacts. The first decision the shy teen must make is who he or she wants to date. Shy teens are often attracted to their most popular classmates. Perhaps he is drawn to people he feels can carry the conversation for him, or perhaps she is fantasizing in a Cinderella way. It is helpful to have your child think realistically about who interests him and what attracts him to that person.

One way to get to the bottom of the question of who to date is to have your shy teen draw a large circle on a piece of paper. Have her put her own name in the middle of the circle. Within the circle, have her write the names of the people she would like to ask out, placing those who are likely to say yes closer to her name, those likely to say no further away.

When your teen has a few names of people who might go out on a date with her, help her think about the kinds of cues a person gives when they want to show that they like someone. Remember: Poor social appraisal is a hallmark of shyness. Talk about the behaviors your teen should look for: a boy who seeks her out to ask how she is doing; one who "happens" to be there when she gets out of class; one who teases her gently or asks for or gives help with homework. Discuss, also, the ways she might show interest. She might do the teasing, call with a question about homework, pass a silly note.

How to Ask. Once your teen has decided who to ask based on what reasonably seems to be a mutual attraction, he needs to plan how he is going to ask. He should know that this is a sweaty-palms time for even the most outgoing teenager. To make it a successful experience for a shy teen, he must plan ahead.

As he talks about where he wants to take his date, and how he will ask, be sure to ask him how he thinks he might feel, and what his thoughts will be as he is asking. He will no doubt feel anxious, and his self-talk might be extremely negative—so negative, in fact, that he might not be able to ask her out at all. The feelings of anxiety will start when he talks it through with you. That is good. He needs to accustom himself to the anxious, uncomfortable feeling, so that when it hits during the real thing it is not so bothersome.

Have your shy teen practice asking someone out on a date until he can do it without nervousness. He can practice in front of the mirror, work with a parent, or talk to the dog. The more he rehearses, the easier it will be. If he is open to role-playing, you should take the role of your child, and have him take the role of the person he wants to date. Be sure to include scenarios that may be disastrous, such as asking out a girl who is surrounded by her friends, and having her friends giggle and tease. Have some versions of the scenario play out well, while others should be silly and lighthearted. Ask if your teen thinks that writing a note would be a good way to avoid the possible humiliation of a face-to-face encounter. (It isn't. Ask what would happen if the note fell into the wrong hands!)

Rejection and Back-up Plans. Everybody gets turned down, even the most popular kid in school. Your shy teen must be prepared for this possibility. The best defense is a good offense: Plan B and Plan C and Plan D. If the first person turns him down, he should have the name of someone else he would like to ask out.

It is important to interject a note of reality into dating. Help your teen come to the realization that if she gets turned down for a date, the world will not stop spinning. This does not mean to dismiss the real pain that rejection can cause, but to keep it in a realistic context.

Planning the Date. Shy adolescents cannot leave anything to chance. Planning ahead is one of the most powerful tools they have. Planning reduces surprises and increases the chances that the date will go well. Shy kids are great catastrophizers; they can easily imagine the things that can go wrong on a date. Conversely, they are great fantasizers who can work out every magical detail on a dream date well in advance. They need some reality checks whether their scenarios are worst-case or best-case. You can help brainstorm alternatives, or responses when things don't go as planned. What if the movie theater is sold out; what if dinner costs more than he planned; what if he wants to go home early.

Have your shy teen plan in advance how he or she wants the date to end. Whether it ends with a handshake, hug, or kiss on the front porch depends on your family values and the chemistry of the date. It is much better for your teen to think about this ahead of time, and to look for cues from his date so that the conclusion of the date is acceptable to both. A successful closure of a date is as important as a good beginning, because it sets up the shy teen for the next date.

Don't let the planning get too mechanical. If your teen seems to fret about the details, or mentions bringing his notes on the date, you'll know it is time to pull back a bit and reintroduce the concept of fun into the preparations. Try to get your child to smile; it relaxes the body and relieves stress.

Debriefing. When the date is over, make time to have your shy teen share some of the details with you. He or she might not care to let you in on either the perceived success or the failures. But if you think you can get a response, your tone should be mildly interested. Your concern is to have your shy teen evaluate an intensely social situation, looking for what she did well, recounting her thoughts and actions, and deciding how to act the next time.

COMPUTERS

Advances in technology and the development of the World Wide Web offer what may look like limitless, safe social interaction possibilities for shy teens. When you encourage your high school student to spend more time with others, she may argue that she spends time chatting on the Internet, or corresponding via e-mail. Some shy teens substitute playing games on the Web for playing games with people. Role-playing games based in fantasy worlds, where the teens get to assume new personalities, are particularly attractive.

If computers attract your child, you may have to be proactive in helping him or her avoid hiding in cyberspace. Inasmuch as you are still the parent in the house, you can set limits on computer time so that it does not take the place of time spent with people.

The Internet can be a useful tool, but shy adolescents can actually do themselves harm if the Internet becomes a social substitute. Recent studies have shown that adolescents often present their ideal selves in chat rooms and with individuals, giving themselves new names and personalities in an attempt to feel more comfortable. But they may not be willing to acknowledge that other people are doing the same thing, and that makes them vulnerable to disappointment, or worse. It is well documented that predatory adults disguise themselves online and seek out lonely teens. In some cases, this practice has led to abusive and dangerous situations when a meeting has been arranged. Shy people can be naive about social situations; they are quick to fantasize and slow to learn.

Time spent on the computer means time not spent with other people. It also may mean time spent forming potentially unpleasant or dangerous relationships. But banning your shy teen from the computer is not the answer. It is an overreaction. The forbidden fruit tastes sweetest, and he will find access to a computer at a library or a café or when you are sleeping. It is better to negotiate with your teen and come up with time limits and usage guidelines that everyone can live with. Be honest about your concerns both for her social life and about the risks involved in forming cyber-relationships. A good tip is to trade one hour of computer time for one hour of a truly social activity, such as a martial arts class or time spent in a committee meeting. And let your child know you are interested in what she's doing on the computer by asking about the conversations she's been having.

THE DAILY DISCUSSION

By the time your shy child is fourteen years old, she is ready for longer discussions with you. (You may find, of course, that other activities interfere with daily discussions, but you should continue to schedule them regularly; certainly no less than once a week.) You can expand your discussion from fifteen minutes to a half hour or an hour. Remember: *The daily discussion is* not *the time to interrogate or lecture*. This is the time to key in on what you have in common with your child, to listen to her explore her emerging passions and opinions, and to relax around her.

As you enjoy your discussions, and if your child feels safe and comfortable, he will begin to open up and share the troubling scenarios caused by his shyness. It might be painful for you to hear stories of his being excluded, rejected, teased, or harassed. Teenagers sometimes use language that sounds harsh or vulgar to parents. In order for your teenager to trust you enough to share openly, you may need to acquiesce to his way of using language. The period when children express their inner feelings best in jargon, slang, and even profanity is usually a passing phase.

When your teen shares a painful incident, the temptation is to sympathize or to rush in with a suggestion on how to fix the problem. This will not help your shy teen, though it may make you feel better. Put on your poker face and use your best listening skills.

Avoid saying "I understand," or "I've been in your shoes," or "I know how you feel." She won't believe you. Even if you were a shy teenager, even if you see direct connections between your life and the life of your child, your child does not want to think that you know what she is feeling. Remember that she is in the business of individuating from you during this period. Letting her talk about her problems is one way to keep her attached in a healthy way. Trying to convince her that you understand her completely might scare her. She needs you to be her parent and not her best friend. To take her feelings on yourself can even have the unintentional effect of invalidating your child's experience.

Your shy teenager's traumatic social experiences or negative self-appraisal may be unexpectedly upsetting to you. It is important to avoid showing your own emotions because that is likely to upset your child. She needs a parent who can listen with a clear head and help her move to a constructive position to learn new skills. Your show of emotion may cause her to shift to a position of comforting and protecting you, in effect, to parent her own parent. If she sees that by being honest she hurts you, she may stop telling you what is going on in her life.

Your shy teenager is talking to you because he trusts you and he wants some help. You must frame your helpful responses in a way that the teenager will accept.

Admit Your Limits. Say "I can't even pretend to know what you are feeling," or "I can't imagine what that must be like." Teenagers have a finely tuned sense of hypocrisy and dishonesty. If you admit that you cannot understand all of their feelings, you are being honest, and you acknowledge that their situation is complex. You avoid erecting barriers or throwing your shy child off-track by making him angry or frustrated with you. When you are honest and genuinely interested in learning what is going on in your child's life, he will want to keep talking.

Avoid the Generation Gap. The generation gap yawns between you and your child the first time you say, "When I was your age . . .". It doesn't matter how you worked out anxiety issues way back when. As far as most teenagers are concerned, whatever happened to you happened in a different age on another planet, and it cannot have any possible relevance to life today. This does not mean that your experience is useless.

Quite the contrary; you may have important tips to share with your child, especially if you were shy at the same age.

The trick is to present your experience in a frame or context that is acceptable to your adolescent. Use opening phrases such as "Someone at work said . . ." "I heard that . . ." or "I saw someone on television who . . .". By removing yourself and your personal experience from the discussion, you increase the chances your teenager will listen. Putting your advice in an acceptable context makes it easier for your shy teenager to listen and learn without having to feel defensive.

Keep It Brief. Fewer words are always better when dealing with any teenager, shy or outgoing. This is a difficult piece of advice for most parents to take. When you are angry or frustrated, it is easy to launch into a tirade. When you are concerned about your shy teenager, it is hard to restrain yourself from going on and on and on about how to fix his problem.

Keep the adult images of the Charlie Brown cartoons in mind. Whenever they spoke, their words came across to the children in a droning blur of sound. That is what your precious words of wisdom sound like if you jabber on too long. Keep it simple, keep it brief.

Adolescent Self-Talk

Teenagers sometimes use raw, shocking language or present their world to us in a way that seems distorted and completely unrealistic. If you can recall, adolescence can be an agonizing and painful time for even the most outgoing, best-adjusted teen. Shy kids struggle through excruciating dilemmas, and they don't always use polite language to talk about it. If your child is expressing his feelings in terms that seem negative and harsh to you, try to relax. If you react too much to the language your teen uses, you cannot help him deal with the anxiety and anger that provoked the choice of words.

Pay attention to his choice of words without judging the language. What you are hearing is his self-talk. This is the voice your shy teen hears. What would you feel like if someone said those kinds of things to you all day? A six-year-old child's self-talk may be "You dummy. Nobody wants to play with you." A sixteen-year-old's is considerably more dramatic and intense, "You idiot. That was the stupidest thing to do. They don't want to talk to you. They don't know you exist. You're ugly and you don't belong here. You're an alien. You're gross." Shy teens can be extremely hard on themselves.

You cannot command a teen to change his self-talk. You might as well tell the tide not to come in. You can influence it, though, by focusing on your shy teen's positive qualities and praising his successes. Make sure that he has incremental, small goals to accomplish and pay attention when he reaches his goals. Give your child the opportunity to do something well every day. Your voice, full of love and admiration, will help to counter the negative self-talk.

If you have been working with your shy child for a while on his shyness issues, then it will be easier to discuss things like negative self-talk. Try to keep the conversation brief and light. Remind your child of techniques that have worked in the past: identifying negative self-talk, changing it to neutral language, relaxing the body, working to positive self-talk. (See Chapter 2.) If you are just beginning to cope with shyness issues, and if your child is open to talking with you about them, you can introduce the concept of self-talk and begin to help him understand how destructive it can be.

Music can play an interesting role at this age. Some people unconsciously choose songs to hum or run through their minds that have lyrics which take on the role of self-talk. Pay attention to this phenomenon in yourself; then bring up the subject with your shy teen. It helps if you know the music she is listening to and can comment on it in a nonjudgmental way.

SCRIPTWRITING, REWRITING, ROLE-PLAYING, AND REHEARSING

Like middle school students, many shy adolescents are leery of highly structured sessions of scriptwriting or role-playing. If you push the issue, you may hear that the idea is "dumb" or "babyish." Your shy teenager still needs the kind of lessons that he can learn from scriptwriting and role-playing; indeed, the highly charged social atmosphere of high school makes planning for social situations and practicing them vitally important.

While some teens will respond to an invitation to rehearse alternatives to a troublesome scenario (these tend to be teens who have worked openly on their shyness issues when they were younger), others will dig in their heels and refuse. A successful parent is a crafty parent. You must be subtle, planning your conversation in advance, scattering clues and concepts in such a way that your teen can't help but be intrigued and pulled into the ideas.

Your maturing teenager will likely prefer to work with one parent on shyness issues, even if he worked with both parents when he was younger. A boy will most likely prefer to work with his mother, while a girl might prefer to work with her father. As children develop into adolescents, they begin to value the opinion of their opposite gender parent more highly. They may be more open to working with the parent of the opposite gender because they want to learn how "the other half" thinks and feels.

Obviously, this will not work in family situations where the parent of the opposite gender is abusive or is peripheral to the child's life. A father who has worked seventy hours a week ever since his daughter was a baby will not be able to connect with her instantly. A mother who has never been part of her son's life will not be able to understand what motivates him or how to listen closely when he needs to unburden himself. No parent who has a pattern of physically or emotionally abusing their shy child will have the kind of trust bond necessary to work through the difficult issues of a shy adolescent.

TEASING

Many parents, particularly fathers, make teasing a big part of the way they relate to their children. This seems all in fun when children are younger. By the time a shy child has grown into adolescence, teasing may get in the way of a supportive relationship with the teasing parent. The teenager will be reluctant to open up about his feelings or to share difficult social situations because he knows it will just result in more teasing. The teasing parent may be disappointed by this turn of events, or he might become defensive and declare that it is all in fun. It's not funny to be teased when you are already hurting.

Techniques

The techniques below can help shy teens take control of their negative self-talk, evaluate the situations that provoke anxiety in them, and develop a tolerance for stressful situations. Share these techniques during teachable moments, those windows of time when you know your shy teen is listening and open to your suggestions. Keep the moment brief and your instruction casual.

Shaping the Right Response. Heather was a shy sixteen-year-old who flat-out refused to use the telephone. She never knew what to say when someone called; the brief silences in a conversation hung for hours in her mind. Just the sound of a ringing phone was enough to waken the butterflies in her stomach and make her palms sweat.

Heather's father knew she needed to plan out her phone conversations ahead of time. He also knew that a direct suggestion from him would likely be dismissed by his daughter. Instead, he took her to the movies and out for ice cream after.

While they ate their hot fudge sundaes, Heather's father brought up the subject of actors. He wondered if they were allowed to make up what they wanted to say while the cameras were rolling. Heather laughed and said no, they had to stick to the script that was written for them. Her father asked if they had to memorize the whole script and shoot every scene in one take. Heather explained what she knew about actors learning their lines. Her father ate his ice cream. He wisely waited for his daughter to make the connection on her own, knowing that was the most powerful way for the lesson to be learned.

Heather mused that maybe she should write out a script

for a phone call. If she had something to read from, maybe she wouldn't be so nervous. Her father agreed and they had a fun time brainstorming the logical and ridiculous things that might happen while she was on the phone, as well as her responses.

This type of covert instruction is called "prompting" or "shaping." It comes from the fact that teens learn best when they come to realizations on their own. It's the difference between feeding a hungry man or teaching him how to fish. You don't have all the answers, and even if you did, your children wouldn't listen to them. Your job is to help nudge your shy teen into finding out the answers herself.

Stimulus Generalization. If the student who sits behind your teenager kicks his seat every day at 2:00 P.M., he will soon begin to feel anxious as soon as he walks in the classroom at 1:35. He has moved from the simple anxiety response of the seat kicking to a larger stimulus generalization of simply entering that particular classroom. It is likely that his anxiety interferes with his ability to listen to the teacher. Even his homework in that class may be hampered because of the physical and emotional stress responses he feels when he approaches the subject. The bully's actions have tainted an entire subject for your shy child.

Shy children might develop multiple triggers like this that get pulled throughout each day. They can make life extremely hard to manage. The first thing to do is to help your teen identify those events or potential events that trigger anxiety. If chemistry class is a trial, is it because of the teacher or something about the classroom? Is he afraid of being called on? Do other people in the class make him nervous? One person in particular? A-ha! You have found the root. Now let your teen explore how that one person's actions have poisoned the classroom.

Identifying the problem is only the first step. It is not enough to think rationally about a problem. Shy adolescents are great thinkers. They must learn to act.

Tell your teen to change his behavior pattern in the classroom that is causing problems. If the problem is the seat-kicker, suggest that he sit in a different seat, away from the bully. If necessary, have him enter the class at the last minute, or arrive first thing to ensure that the bully cannot sit near him. He can get up from his seat to sharpen his pencil or consult a reference book. He needs to break the bonds he has formed between that room, the bully, and his feelings of anxiety.

Heather, in the earlier example, was too scared to talk on the phone. Just the sound of a ringing telephone could make her hands sweat. She also found that if she was reading a book and the phone rang, she became anxious when she picked up the book again. She had generalized her anxious feelings from the phone to include the book.

Heather learned to control her negative self-talk and confront her anxiety response with action. When the phone rang, the first thing she did was to use thought stopping, saying "Stop. Stop. Stop. Stop," until she felt more in control. Then she thought, "I can do this. I can do this." She got up from whatever she was doing and changed her actions for a few minutes. This prevented her from developing multiple triggers for anxiety.

Relaxation Strategies. You can be more specific and open with teenagers about relaxation techniques than you can with younger children. Teenagers have a better sense of the abstract and most are eager to explore the mind-body connection.

The starting point to all relaxation strategies is breathing from the diaphragm. The goal is not deep breathing, but slow, rhythmic breathing, like waves rolling in from the ocean. Look for magazine articles that describe breathing techniques that you can share with your shy teen. You can also buy relaxation tapes or CDs that your shy teen can listen to on a Walkman.

Many adolescents are intrigued by meditation and yoga. Look for classes in these techniques; enroll both your shy teen and yourself. The relaxation strategies that are so helpful for shy teens work just as well for stressed parents of shy teens. Enrolling in the class together will develop a common interest and give you a chance to enjoy each other's company while learning something new.

The relaxation response is a direct contrast to the anxiety response that controls so much of a shy child's life. They cannot coexist in your child's mind. Once your shy teen is familiar and comfortable with relaxation techniques, encourage her to use them in anxiety-provoking situations. Use them yourself as you prepare for a stressful meeting or confront a difficult person and report back to your teen. Ask for her advice. Your shy teen will learn by teaching you, just as you learn from teaching her.

Journal Writing. Keeping a journal is an invaluable exercise for shy teenagers. A journal is a terrific place to unload anxiety and pour out feelings that cannot be shared with anyone else. Journals don't judge.

Try to persuade your child to keep a journal by buying one for her and then by suggesting a time during each evening that is exclusively for writing. If you are successful, your child is the one who must decide whether or not to share her journal with you. You must respect her limits. As long as you do not suspect that your child is suicidal, the journal is off-limits. If you snoop and she finds out, you will have broken the most important bond of trust your shy child has with you.

When your teenager runs into a social situation that causes him trouble, be sure to encourage him to write about it in his journal. If he shares the journal entry with you, you may feel that he has exaggerated the situation on paper: "As I tripped over my shoelace, the entire student body turned to stare. One thousand faces laughed at me, one thousand fingers pointed. I am so humiliated I can never go back to the auditorium." Your shy teenager's journal will provide you with stunning examples of the extreme drama he experiences in his self-talk.

If your adolescent regularly shares her journal with you, encourage her to go through older journal entries and circle words or phrases of negative self-talk. Have her write a neutral or positive self-talk message to balance the negative. Then ask her to rate how believable the neutral or positive messages are, and to rate the probability of using one of the new statements. Keep working with her until she comes up with a useful statement that she can believe in and use.

When to Hug

In the course of subtly guiding your shy teenager to rehearse difficult social situations or changing negative self-talk to positive, things may get emotional. Do not be surprised if talking about shyness issues or practicing scenarios cause an unexpected outburst. It may come out as rage or sadness; your teenager may holler or dissolve into tears. This can be a very good sign; your shy adolescent is reliving the kind of anxiety that he suffers through in social situations.

You might be tempted to hug or comfort if your teenager cries, or reprimand if he uses foul language in his frustration. Hold back. Listen intently. If you rush in with hugs and tissues, or a disapproving lecture about swear words, you will not help. Rescuing him from his emotions will cause more damage.

Your teenager is experiencing the same high anxiety level that he experiences during awkward social situations. He must develop a harder shell. Let him talk it out. Let him brainstorm alternative ways to deal with the situation. Help him examine his self-talk.

The time for hugs and comfort is after your child has plotted out a constructive alternative to dissolving in tears or running away. At that point, he has taken control of his anxiety. If he still needs comforting, this is when you can offer a hug.

CHAPTER SUMMARY

1. There are plenty of positive things about living with a teenager, but developmental changes make it harder to discuss shyness issues.

2. Parents need to maintain contact with school officials when their shy teen is in high school, and allow the teen to assume more responsibility gradually for planning.

3. Shy teens often need to develop basic social skills.

4. It is not a crime to graduate from high school without

ever going out on a date. If a teenager does make plans to date, planning out how to arrange it and where to go will help make the date more successful.

5. Shy teens should not substitute time on the computer for true social interactions.

6. Parents must resist the impulse to lecture during the daily discussion period.

7. Role-playing, scriptwriting, and rehearsing must be more subtle with teens.

8. Parents must allow their teens to work through their feelings of anxiety instead of trying to shelter them from anything uncomfortable.

Chapter 10

SETTING THE SHY CHILD FREE

You and your shy child have survived play groups, first grade, the cafeteria, bullies, thoughtless teachers, cruel cliques, school dances, class presentation disasters, gym class nightmares, dates, no dates, hormones, and broken hearts. You have celebrated the first time she greeted a friend, raised her hand to ask a question, found a caring teacher, spoke up to defend herself, talked on the phone, tried out for a team, went on a sleep-over, played the solo, presented a project in front of the class, belonged to a group, came through college interviews with flying colors. It is time for your shy child to leave home. You are quietly proud or utterly terrified. Or both.

Letting go of a shy child can be difficult, both because of parental anxiety about what the child faces and the strong bonds between shy child and parent. Some families unwittingly encourage dependency even after their child is an adult. In an attempt to protect her, they make it too easy for her to remain at home.

The years after your child leaves high school call for you to maintain a strong connection—but at a distance. Your child must find his own way, be it through college or in the workplace. He must know that he can come home if he needs to. But he needs to know you trust him with decisions about his future.

"LAST CHANCE" TRAP

Families who have not earlier confronted the issue of shyness with a child sometimes make drastic and unwise decisions when that child prepares to leave home. During a shy child's last year of high school, parents suddenly become Cassandras, making dire predictions about all the bad things that will happen if he does not learn how to "get over" his shyness. Their intentions are good; they are trying to prepare their child for the expectations and pressures of the adult world. However, the technique is inefficient at best, and harmful at worst. The implication that an individual has no hope for a satisfactory future unless he becomes an outgoing person can, in the worst-case scenario, become a self-fulfilling prophecy.

When such families arrive at a therapist's office, they are usually there for the quick fix. A therapist may decide to spend six or eight sessions with the parents alone, where he will discuss their unrealistic expectations of their child and to help them to focus on and accentuate the positive attributes of their shy child. It is a challenge for parents, those who have waited until high school, to restrain themselves from berating their child about socialization issues. They have to learn that their child has been beating *himself* up about these issues for years.

NIGHTMARE OF COMMUNICATION

Even for parents who have helped their child reduce social anxieties since early childhood, the transition from high school student to college student or independent adult can be difficult. High school seniors are notorious for their unwillingness to take advice. Just at the time when you are ready to pass on the wisdom you have gained from your own life experiences, your child stops listening. Take the child's independent streak, add parental anxieties, throw in a dash of insecurity about how to pay for college or find a paying job, and you have a communication nightmare—even with your children who are not shy.

It is important to remain clear about the ultimate goal for this age, which is to help your shy child find his or her *own* path in life and develop the social skills and self-confidence he or she will need to be happy. You cannot force a person to be outgoing, and there is no reason to suppose that being outgoing is necessary for your child to live a fulfilling life.

If you find yourself mired in worries about how your child will fare out in the world, assign yourself and your shy child small goals. Go out to breakfast and enjoy a relaxed conversation that does not touch on any of the sensitive issues that plague you both. When you are rested, relaxed, and ready to listen, ask what your child sees in his future. When you show respect and honor his desires, it is easier for him to listen to your advice and concerns. When your advice and concerns are expressed in the context of his vision for himself, then there is much more potential for a satisfying exchange of information.

COLLEGE

Your role in your child's college career is not limited to paying the bills. You can add your voice to the many that will be calling out to your child as she tries to decide which college to go to. But for the college experience to be successful, which college she goes to *must*, finally, be your child's choice. If you pressure a shy child into going to a school where she is not comfortable, there is every likelihood that she will—consciously or unconsciously—sabotage your decision.

By starting early—in your child's junior or senior year—you can go to colleges with enough time on your hands to let him get a real feel for each one. Many families set aside the summer between the junior and senior years to visit as many colleges as possible. Beginning with colleges that are nearby your home, give your shy child a taste of college life by visiting campuses nearby and eating lunch in the cafeteria, or shopping in the bookstore. Set up meetings with the high school guidance counselor who is in charge of disseminating information about colleges, and make sure your child has a comfortable relationship with him or her. As you discuss options with your child, give him the option of attending schools close to home as well as those far away, but try to convince him to live on campus if possible.

Be aware that your shy child feels torn between his yearning for independence and his anxiety about living away from you. Your calm demeanor and support will make his decision easier. Refrain from becoming either too maudlin or too celebratory about the child leaving home. This is a matter-of-fact transition, both for the child and the family. Shy college students feel the most free to blossom at school when their family roots are nourished and healthy.

Don't neglect the role of siblings. Shy kids are frequently quite close to their siblings, and can experience a surprising sense of loss when they move away from home. Parents need to honor that special bond and create opportunities for the shy child and her siblings to maintain their relationship when separated. Give your shy child a special phone card for sibling calls, or encourage e-mail correspondence. Take the time to help the stay-at-home child prepare care boxes for the college student, and brainstorm with the college student about what she may send home to the sibling.

A Positive Transition

Erica's parents did a magnificent job helping their shy daughter transition from high school to college. Erica set the course by choosing the colleges she was interested in. The family planned well in advance, visited the colleges, and gave her the information and support she needed to make her decision.

Once Erica was accepted, her parents maintained a cheerful, positive approach. They did not bog her down with horror stories of their own college years, or dire predictions about the amount of work she would have to do. They let her enjoy the summer and helped her prepare for the big move.

When it came time to move Erica to college, her family was ready. She had packed several things from home to help make her dorm room a familiar and comfortable place. The family and campus volunteers helped carry everything from the Jeep up to her room, but her parents did not unpack or organize Erica's room. That was something for Erica to do with her roommates; it would provide a great icebreaking opportunity.

Erica and her parents went for a leisurely stroll around

campus. They arranged to rent her a refrigerator; they walked over to the work-study office where Erica would later sign up for a job. They had lunch together. After lunch, they went to the library to see about reserving a study carrel for Erica. She had decided to sign up for a quad room (four roommates living together), and recognized that there would be times when she needed quiet solitude to recharge her internal batteries. The library offered a safe, practical haven. When they went back to the dormitory, Erica's roommates had arrived and her resident assistant was there. Erica's parents talked to the RA and wrote down her number, just in case. Then they took a deep breath, kissed their daughter goodbye, and left. They would call on Sunday.

It was a poignant day, and sad in many ways for her parents, but they stayed positive and upbeat. By staying in the background as Erica explored the campus, they offered their shy child some much needed structure, comfort, and a feeling of connection during a stressful day. The campus tour served much the same function as when they took Erica into her elementary school the week before kindergarten started.

Roommates and the Need for Solitude

The decision about roommates is usually made while your child is still living at home during his last year of high school. If your child has signed up for a suite with two, three, or four roommates, that is a marvelous start. We discussed the pros and cons of living with one roommate versus being part of a larger crowd. The most difficult challenge presented by the larger group is your child's need for solitude.

You may hear your child complain about the noise level in the room, the irritation that he is never alone, or his roommates' habits. Your child needs to put some regular alone time back into his life. The good news about college for shy people is that it is a twenty-four-hour-a-day social experience. It becomes the bad news if the shy student cannot claim some time every day for himself. Shy college students require a period of precious isolation during which they can reduce their stimulation overload and recenter themselves.

UNEXPECTED INFLUENCES

Help your shy college student evaluate what influences her own behavioral patterns. For example, if she goes to a school in a different part of the country, changes in weather and sunlight may have an effect on her mood. There have not been any studies linking seasonal affective disorder (SAD) to shy people, but students who are hypersensitive may react more to environmental changes. Frustrations with living conditions and roommates may be influenced by unsuspected culprits like the weather.

Make sure that your child has realistic expectations of his roommates. If he has trouble, encourage him to talk to his resident assistant or other people on the floor to gain perspective. Is there an objective concern about the roommate's behavior, or is your child reacting in a more sensitive way to normal behavior. It is rare for students to be allowed to change roommates in the middle of a semester; dealing with unpleasant people is an unfortunate fact of life. Encourage your shy student to seek out friends in social clubs, sports teams, or other campus activities. When it comes time to register for the next year's housing, his goal should be to have a group of friends he wants to live with.

Classes

There are a few bits of sideline advice you can give your shy student that will help make scheduling classes and the mechanics of campus life easier. It's best not to be too forceful with this advice, but at moments when you think she is ready to listen to your suggestions, here are some things she can think about. She might not agree with you, or she may make a show of dismissing your advice, but when she is standing alone on a campus of ten thousand strangers, she might remember what you said.

- *Find a mentor.* Shy students rarely develop interpersonal relationships with their high school teachers, but they need to know how important a mentoring relationship with a responsible professor can be both during the college years and later. Most colleges appoint a professor to oversee each incoming student's schedule. Help your child find out how flexible this system is. Encourage her to change advisors if she's uncomfortable with the one assigned to her. She should listen to older students, and seek a professor who is familiar with her field of study and is approachable. Since your child will most likely be reticent about "bothering" her teachers, let her know that most teachers appreciate students who make an effort to develop a student-mentor relationship outside the classroom. It is one reason they have chosen teaching as a profession.

- *Make your schedule fit your lifestyle.* Help your child evaluate his own body clock. Will an 8:00 A.M. statistics course work for a night owl? Should an early bird register for a 6:00 P.M. graduate course? You cannot choose your child's classes, but you can encourage him to keep his personality in mind. He needs to think through his course decisions, particularly in the first year, when he will be coping with transition stress.

- *Plan ahead!* Many schools offer students the opportunity to register for classes early if they volunteer to work during the registration and orientation period. Volunteering early in the semester is a terrific way to meet people as well as to provide more scheduling flexibility.

Work-Study

Work-study is wonderful for shy college students. Some parents worry about forcing their child to work at college, and are prepared to sacrifice so that their child only has to think about making good grades and making friends. Grades are often not a problem for a shy student. But to make friends, he often needs structure. The working environment for college students almost always involves working with other people— in the library, the cafeteria, the gym. Work-study forces shy students into social settings. His self-talk might convince him to miss the Literature Club meeting time after time, but if he doesn't show up for his shift in the bookstore, there are consequences. Be sure that he chooses a work-study job that surrounds him with people; no lonely security guard shifts.

Earning money at school also gives the shy student a sense of responsibility that builds self-confidence. Earning money is a wonderful secondary reinforcer. When a student works to pay for his education, he becomes more vested in his own success. The hours required by work-study also force shy students to plan ahead and structure their research and study time. Outgoing college students constantly vent about their frustrations, their problems, and their worries. When your shy student is in a work-study program that puts him in the company of these gregarious extroverts, he'll be relieved to hear that he is not alone with his fears and anxieties.

Extracurricular Activity

Being involved in campus life outside the classroom is just as important for a shy college student as it is for a shy middle school or high school student. Clubs, volunteer groups, a choir, dance troupe, or band are powerful social places where your shy student can find both himself, and friends who may stay with him for life.

Make sure your shy student develops a sense of what activities he wants to sign up for before he arrives on campus. He should be flexible; once school starts he may find he feels more comfortable with the kids who run the coffeehouse than the Astronomy Club. But just as you insisted he participate in middle school and high school, he must leave for college with the understanding that his life must be more than books and solitude.

Encourage your shy student to include some physical activity in her mix of extracurricular activities. She doesn't have to try out for a team, but she can enjoy playing intramural sports, or sign up for racquetball or tennis matches at the gym. Depending on the school, there may be new, exotic activities such as crew, tai chi, or boxing. Your shy child must reconnect with her body several times a week. It will draw her out of the overactive imagination, and keep her healthy and strong.

OVERCOMMITMENT AND THE NEED TO BE ASSERTIVE

Shy college students who take the plunge into social activities can sometimes find themselves miserably unhappy, not because of social anxiety, but because they have taken on too much. In their search for a degree of social acceptance, they'll say yes to everything. "Sure, I'll set up for the party; I'd be happy to organize that fund-raiser; count on me to get five hundred signatures on the petition." They can't say no because they don't know how to say it in a way that feels socially appropriate. When they become overwhelmed, they feel as though they have let their new friends down, and all the old negative self-talk crashes down around them. They withdraw, shut down. They make excuses. In the worst cases students have left school rather than face up to the commitments they can't keep.

Shy people often benefit from assertiveness training. They can sign up for a course, read some books about it, or discuss with you the necessity for saying no, and the many ways it can be done. A great technique is to stall. Encourage your shy student to say "I need to check my calendar in my room," or "I think I'm busy already." They must learn that it is socially acceptable to turn someone down. "Thanks for thinking of me, but I can't help right now. I'm flattered you thought of me, but I already have too much on my plate this semester." (If your shy student can hear you gracefully declining volunteer work before she leaves home, she'll have a great model to work from.)

Throwing in the Towel

What if your shy college student is on the phone in tears every night for weeks on end? Or the college contacts you, with the news that your child has yet to turn up for a class? How does a parent know when to step in?

Many young adults go through a period of transitional grief the first few weeks of school. If your student is still highly anxious and emotional after the first month, then you should consider visiting him. Don't quiz him. Don't threaten or lecture. Take him out to dinner, away from campus. Spend Saturday together on campus, away from his dorm. Go to a movie. Hold your tongue and listen, listen, listen. Try to get him to evaluate the root causes of his anxiety. Is he lonely for a friend? Does the amount of studying overwhelm him? Is he having a hard time adjusting to the physical environment of the campus? Does the requirement of large group gatherings, such as eating in the cafeteria or attending a large seminar class, stress him?

If at all possible, try to get your child to finish the semester. The feeling of accomplishment of sticking it out that long will be important, plus he may have adjusted by the end of the marking period. Plan for what he will do after he leaves the campus. The best alternative is attending a smaller school closer to home, preferably one where he can live on campus. If you feel, and he agrees, that he is completely overwhelmed, then enroll him in a community college and welcome him back home with love and understanding. The maxim of small steps still applies to college-age shy adults.

Above all, don't judge, condemn, express disappointment, or holler. If your child cannot adjust comfortably to college, it is not a reflection on you.

DATING

It is impossible to overestimate how important dating becomes after high school. During the college years and those first years in the workforce, many people in our culture find marriage partners or enjoy long-term relationships that are significant. Yet for shy young adults, developing interpersonal relationships is the most difficult and anxiety-producing task before them. Dating issues bring more shy young adults into the offices of therapists than any other concern.

The same types of social anxieties that haunt shy kids in high school continue to make dating difficult later. But in high school, there might have been plenty of kids who didn't date. Now it seems as though everyone does it. And worse, they seem to date easily, laughing, touching, knowing how to say the right thing, never making the wrong move.

The tensions may be compounded for some by confusion about their sexual identity. Some shy young adults interpret their difficulty in getting dates or their reluctance even to try as proof they are homosexual. Confusion about sexual identity is not uncommon and does not last forever. Whether parents like to acknowledge it or not, college, especially, can be a time for sexual exploration. People who go on to lead heterosexual lives may have homosexual relationships, and those who later lead homosexual lives may have heterosexual relationships.

The distance between your home and the emerging adult who is your child prohibits you from meddling in his or her love life. It is none of your business until and unless your child chooses to talk about it. If you try to make it your business, constantly asking for details or teasing about dates, those phone calls home will become brief.

Respect your child's privacy, but be ready to offer support if she asks for it. With your child at the age she is, you can offer stories of your own awkward first dates. Explain that not everyone is an expert on love by age twenty-one.

WHEN TO CALL THE PROFESSIONALS

During the years from age seventeen to twenty-five severe mental illness may present itself. Your child's introverted nature does not put him any more at risk for disabling mental conditions than the general population. But this is the time when serious conditions can develop, for reasons that are not yet clear to medical science.

Shy teenagers and young adults *are* at increased risks for slipping into depression when they leave home. If they did not actively participate in the decisions surrounding where to go to school or what type of job to take, the risk is even greater.

You should consider taking action if you notice any of the following:

- A change in your child's normal hygiene habits;

- Ambivalence about things that were once important;

- Consistently more negative than positive self-assessment. (Keep a pad by the phone. Mark down a plus sign for every good thing your child says about himself and a minus sign for each negative.);

- A distinct downturn in grades;

- Difficulty holding a job; or

- Holing up in a room; refusing to attend class or join any activities.

If you suspect a problem with depression, don't try to fix it over the phone. Plan a weekend visit. Take your child out for dinner and do something together you both enjoy. Get a feel for her mood before you question her directly about your concerns. If you feel uneasy, do not ignore your intuition or the obvious evidence that something is wrong. Consult a professional. Be aware that depression can lead to self-destructive behavior with drugs or alcohol or inappropriate friendships. If you have any suspicions in these areas, don't hesitate to seek help. You may or may not have to work independently of the school in seeking psychological help for your child. In most cases, it is not helpful to count on the facilities of the student mental health department to treat your child effectively.

THE LATE BLOOMER

Shy young adults are famous for being late bloomers. If you were a shy child and didn't come into a strong sense of self-confidence until you were out of high school, then you may be more patient with your shy child. If you have not seen this phenomenon on your own, you may be a nervous wreck by the time your shy student is nineteen years old. Go to any high school reunion—you will find a small group of attractive, confident, successful alumni that make the rest of the class shake their heads, "Do you remember how shy they were back then?" You have found the late bloomers.

For these shy students, college is a ticket to paradise. It's their second chance at social acceptance without the hormonal attacks of early adolescence. The cast-iron cliques of high school have dissolved. The larger canvas of college means there are more chances for a shy child to find someone with her interests, attitude, and perspective. Everyone is equal in college, and people tend to be more forgiving of personal quirks. Shy college students who are comfortable in their choice of college and have good support from home can relax and finally incorporate friends and interpersonal relationships into their lives. The shy child blooms; the shy child's parents breathe a sigh of relief.

THE LATE REBEL

Not all types of late-blooming behavior are positive. Some parents of shy college students are shocked when their child acts out with negative rebellious behavior. They thought their child had made it through her teenage years without falling into dangerous patterns. Then they get a phone call about their child's binge drinking, drug use, or dangerous sexual behavior. Or their child comes home with body piercings, tattoos, or extreme political or religious views. What happened?

Rebelliousness, in and of itself, is not a bad thing. Shy adolescents are often overcontrolled in high school because they are paralyzed by their fears of social interaction. They are more comfortable in college. They relax to the point where they act out in the ways their peers did three to four years earlier. It scares parents when they see their child rejecting their values, but as long as the child is not acting in a self-destructive or violent way, parents do best to stay on the sidelines. It is each generation's obligation to question the values of its parents. That is how the culture grows.

Rebellion takes on many forms. It sometimes takes place in the gym. Parents who have never thought of their children as athletic are stunned to find out that their son tried out for the soccer team and made it or that their daughter is on her way to setting school records in track. Again, the atmosphere of college, and the developing maturity of the shy student allows the student to try things that she always dreamed of, but was too nervous to try before. They have the confidence to express new interests, sometimes with wonderful results. One young man who did not play sports in high school joined the football team at his community college and developed into such a player that he earned a full football scholarship to Ohio University!

CULTS

Cults represent a real threat to college students who feel isolated and unsure of themselves. This does not necessarily mean that your child is at risk. If you have been working with him to develop his "anxiety callus" and he attends the college of his choice, chances are he will be fine. But all parents must be aware of the danger of cults.

Cults offer a false sense of belonging to students who are lonely. Their claim to have all the answers seduces students feeling overwhelmed by internal questions. They give unconditional acceptance and affiliation to students who feel they do not fit in elsewhere. If you have spent six weeks in your room, afraid to speak to anyone, and as lonely as you have ever been in your whole life, the offer of unlimited access to a group can feel like a lifesaver. But cults or cultlike religious groups often pull in confused young people and make it very difficult for them to disengage. Some have even been accused of brainwashing young adults to the point that they reject their families.

The best defense against cults is a good offense. Do not push your shy young adult to attend the college that you want; let her choose for herself. Plan the transition to college carefully. Keep the lines of communication open regarding her social contacts. Without appearing to be meddling and nosy, make sure your child knows she can talk to you about the friends she is making. Remain in contact with her weekly, and visit her if you feel something is wrong. Most important, take some time before college begins to discuss the issue of cults. Do some research on which ones operate on college campuses and how they tend to approach students. Let your child know what their techniques are so she can be wary if someone uses those techniques with her.

LIFE AFTER COLLEGE

Most shy people find that college life is wonderful. The university is a warm place, accepting of eccentrics and introverts. The emphasis on introspection and analysis is one they feel comfortable with. Shy college students are notorious for not wanting to come home. They find summer internships; they work as dorm counselors. They go to graduate school. They keep going to graduate school. There are some who feel that college professors represent a large group of shy students who found their niche in the academic world.

Parents may worry when their child, particularly a shy introvert, decides to stay on campus. It can shake up the parental timetable. You were expecting at least three more years of having your child home in the summer; then you would really have to say goodbye. The call in early May that informs you that he found a job and is sharing an apartment with a friend for the summer can take your breath away. Don't complain.

Summer jobs or internships offer a terrific stepping-stone to meaningful work after graduation. If your shy student stays on campus in the summer, encourage him to get a job in his field of interest. He may need some help figuring out how to do this: how to approach professors, how to get acquainted with the function of the campus job search coordinator, how to prepare for interviews. The process itself and the work atmosphere of an internship position are excellent ways for shy students to get ready for the work world.

THE WORKING WORLD

Many people experience the workplace as a harsh and cold environment. Shy adults may not find open-minded roommates or soul mates willing to offer a seat in the cafeteria. While high school and college represent a whole way of life, most jobs are means to an end. By the time your shy child enters the workforce, she will be expected to have mastered the social graces and be able to control her anxiety. If she hasn't, she will not be an attractive employee.

Shy people who have not learned how to deal with their social anxieties often choose jobs that require them to work with things instead of people. They seek jobs in such fields as engineering or data analysis. The choice of a career should be an outgrowth of a person's passions and talents. The goal for a shy child, and her parents, is to manage the shyness to the degree that it does not interfere with life goals such as career choice.

Social skills are in the spotlight during the job interview. Shy adults often do quite well in one-on-one interviews, particularly if they are seeking a job that is an outgrowth of one of their interests. A one-on-one situation is structured and easy to prepare for. Unfortunately, many companies are abandoning the one-on-one interview in favor of all-day interviews that involve group meetings and role-plays that mimic daily work environments. Large firms run applicants through psychological screenings and often use a panel interview as part of the hiring process. Shy people need to rehearse endlessly for a panel interview. Many describe it as their worst nightmare. They sit in front of a group of strangers whose sole purpose is to evaluate them. The applicant feels as if all his flaws are on display. Equally terrifying is an interview process in which the applicant is required to give a presentation. If the shy applicant has not learned how to rehearse and manage anxiety, it can feel like the third-grade nightmare come to life. His anxiety defeats him and he doesn't get the job.

Shy people get the job they want when they research and prepare. If they know what to expect from the interview process and they rehearse for it, mentally or with a friend or family member, they can do quite well. Shy adults must remember that strangers project negative qualities onto a blank slate, or a silent newcomer. They must arrive at an interview or the workplace prepared for some small talk and having an established plan of action.

In modern society, social skills are required for all jobs.

Even engineers must know how to deal with customers. If you feel your shy student is deliberately steering down a career path she thinks will keep her away from stressful situations with others, help her research her options. She needs to come to the conclusion, on her own, that all jobs involve interpersonal contact. She can improve her social skills as steadily as she improves her technical skills.

Shy adults must be encouraged to develop a life outside the workplace. Just as when they were students, they must seek out extracurricular activities. This is harder to do outside of an academic setting, so be prepared with suggestions about how they can locate clubs or interest groups. Most towns have activities such as recreational sports teams, fitness centers, and bridge, chess, or card clubs. Encourage your young adult to find out what his peers are doing. Maybe it's time to take up golf but only if your child has an interest in it. If she feels forced by social pressures to do something she wouldn't normally do, it will reactivate those negative thoughts and self-doubt. Her own interests must be her guide.

Shy adults can apply the same lessons to the work world that they applied to their high school or college years. They must be particularly careful not to overcommit, or agree to take on projects or responsibilities they are not prepared for or do not want to do. If your shy adult is flailing in his new role, ask him to review what he absolutely needs to do, and what extras have been foisted on him. He might need to practice saying, "Let me get back to you about that."

DAILY DISCUSSION

When your shy one is away at college or in the world of work, the opportunities for a daily discussion are necessarily limited.

But this important feature of your relationship with your child does not have to end. In fact, both you and your child will be better off if it doesn't.

Establish a time for a weekly phone call. Many people choose Sunday, because that has traditionally been a day when some time is set aside for family. It does not matter which day you choose, but it should be a day and a time when you will always be available to your child. It doesn't matter if he's twenty-two years old and he stands a foot taller than you, or if she's managing stock portfolios and trading commodities, shy adults love knowing there is a time every week when they can touch base with family. As long as you don't use the time to nag or complain, they will look forward to that phone call every week.

Don't be alarmed if you feel that your child regresses during the first few weeks of college or when he has been on the job in another town for a month or two. You may hear reports of immature behavior; there may be tears, declarations of loneliness, a sense of feeling lost. This is normal for the first week or two, but should fade as the shy person orients himself to his surroundings and makes friends. If this behavior persists, or deteriorates into depression, you need to take a trip to assess the situation for yourself.

Chances are you will hear a few bouts of self-doubt and misery, and then the phone calls will become a bit awkward. What is there to talk about after he has settled in? Use those common interests that you've developed over the years; mention a team you both follow or report on your latest adventure in oil painting. Asking if your child needs money is always a popular opening.

Be prepared to hear your child try out new personalities. He might change his career plans or want to change his major every other week. If your child had been oriented toward one set of life goals through high school, this may be a surprise. Do not react or thunder or judge on the telephone. You are listening, and he trusts you enough to share his new dreams and ideas. Let him talk and explore. Encourage him to try different courses—that is what college is for.

Your shy student wants to hear about what is going on at home. Watching parents grow and change comes as a delightful surprise to young adults. Now that you have more free time on your hands, sign up for a class, take up a new exercise, join a poetry group. Explore a passion and tell your shy child about it during your weekly phone call. He will be proud of you, and he'll learn from your great example.

Stay positive. Your goal is to stay connected with your shy student. You want to hear about the food in the cafeteria and the escapades with red socks in the laundry. He'll tell you about his friends and his fears. When it's time for the phone call to end, you should each walk away from the call with a warm glow that will last through the week.

ROLE-PLAYING AND REHEARSING SCENARIOS

It is difficult to participate in role-playing or rehearsing scenarios over the telephone. Not only does it feel silly, but it is not realistic in a manner that will help a young adult. With your child far away, the way she prepares for anxiety-producing social scenarios changes.

Listen carefully during phone calls for what needs to be rehearsed. Ask about your child's friends and the problems he is dealing with. Suggest that your child help out a friend who needs to give a speech or talk to a notoriously cranky professor. Your shy student has a lot of practice in these types of rehearsals. If he is the one who first offers to help, he'll feel more confident when he asks the friend to return the favor.

Send your child books about visualization. The imagination is a powerful tool and your child should know how to harness it for positive ends. Share the scenarios in your life that you are mentally preparing for—a confrontation at work or a painful discussion with your own family members. Remind your shy student of how all her rehearsing in elementary, middle, and high school paid off. She has the tools she needs, and will use them with a little encouragement.

LETTING GO

It is never easy to let go of a child. It may feel impossible to let go of a shy child who needed your guidance, who came to you in tears, who trusted you enough to see his gentle introspective nature. You know how cold the world is. You're afraid he'll be eaten alive.

Nature has a way of dealing with these strong emotions. The natural course of action is for young adults to separate from their parents, and go on to develop their own families. Shy kids follow the same script. When your college student comes home for a break, she may seem like a different person. She *is* a different person. She doesn't live in your house anymore. The sum total of her experiences include things you don't know of, things that she doesn't have to tell you. She might be ornery, haughty, or a pain in the neck. Many parents look forward to that first break with longing, then find that they can't wait for the student to go back to school.

Respect the distance that your college student puts between the two of you. He needs to stretch out, to grow and mature, before he can come back to you. And come back he will. The bonds between a shy child and parent are unusually durable and strong. If you have worked together to help him control his anxiety, you have shared a difficult journey. You have opened up to each other, trusted each other, known pain and joy that other parents never experience.

CHAPTER SUMMARY

1. Don't fall into the "last chance" trap and berate your shy student that if he doesn't become outgoing immediately, he will ruin his life.

2. Let your shy child choose his own college or his post–high school plans.

3. Guide the transition to college in a positive, upbeat manner.

4. Dating is the most important issue to college-age students.

5. Shy students often need assertiveness training to learn how to say no.

6. Shy students succeed when they prepare and rehearse for job interviews and new work situations.

7. Establish a weekly phone call to take the place of your daily discussions.

8. Visit your shy child if you are worried that she is slipping into depression.

ABOUT THE AUTHOR

WARD KENT SWALLOW, PH.D., is the former clinical director of the Department of Pediatric Psychiatry at Children's Hospital Medical Center of Akron and is now in private practice in Las Vegas. The author of numerous papers and articles on shyness, Dr. Swallow has many years of clinical experience with shy children and their parents and is widely regarded as a valued resource for parents seeking reassurance and help.